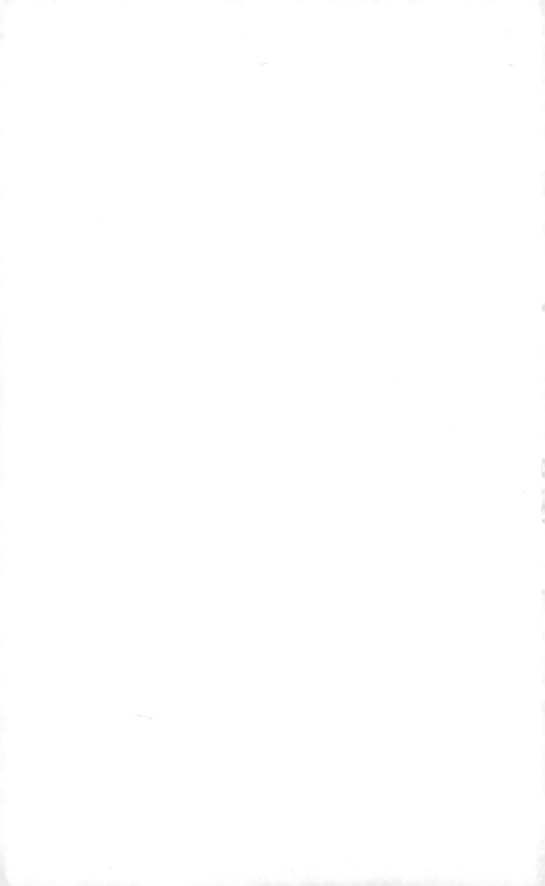

DEPRESSION

**Recent Titles in the
Biographies of Disease Series**

Parkinson's Disease
Nutan Sharma

DEPRESSION

Blaise A. Aguirre

Biographies of Disease
Julie K. Silver, M.D., Series Editor

GREENWOOD PRESS
Westport, Connecticut • London

Library of Congress Cataloging-in-Publication Data

Aguirre, Blaise A.
   Depression / Blaise A. Aguirre.
      p. ; cm.—(Biographies of disease, ISSN 1940-445X)
   Includes bibliographical references and index.
   ISBN-13: 978-0-313-34219-6 (alk. paper)
   1. Depression, Mental. I. Title. II. Series.
   [DNLM: 1. Depression. 2. Adolescent. WM 171 A284d 2008]
   RC537.A384 2008
   616.85'27—dc22   2007048216

British Library Cataloguing in Publication Data is available.

Library of Congress Catalog Card Number: 2007048216
ISBN: 978-0-313-34219-6
ISSN: 1940-445X

First published in 2008

Greenwood Press, 88 Post Road West, Westport, CT 06881
An imprint of Greenwood Publishing Group, Inc.
www.greenwood.com

Printed in the United States of America

The paper used in this book complies with the
Permanent Paper Standard issued by the National
Information Standards Organization (Z39.48–1984).

10 9 8 7 6 5 4 3 2 1

Contents

Series Foreword

Every killer has a story to tell, and so it is with diseases as well: about how it started long ago and began to take the lives of its innocent victims, about the way it hurts us, and about how we are trying to stop it. In this *Biographies of Disease* series, the authors tell the stories of the diseases that we have come to know and fear.

The stories of these killers have all of the components that make for great literature. There is incredible drama played out in real-life scenes from the past, present, and future. You'll read about how men and women of science stumbled trying to save the lives of those they aimed to protect. Turn the pages and you'll also learn about the amazing success of those who fought the killer and won, saving thousands of lives in the process.

If you don't want to be a health professional or research scientist now, when you finish this book you may think differently. The men and women in this book are heroes who often risked their own lives to save ours. This is the biography of a killer, but it is also the story of real people who made incredible sacrifices to stop it in its tracks.

Julie K. Silver, M.D.
Assistant Professor, Harvard Medical School
Department of Physical Medicine and Rehabilitation

Preface

This book on depression is the result of weaving years of clinical and research experience together with the richness of the historical accounts of the illness into a tapestry integrating impersonal and sterile scientific data with familiar and highly personal emotional experiences. The personal stories and the scientific data serve to illuminate each other, and this symbiosis will ultimately lead to a far better understanding of major depression.

An approach to understanding depression that is either purely biological or purely psychological is not helpful. A sole emphasis on "molecular biology" would reduce the depressed brain to a chemically imbalanced organ, denying the profound ways in which the environment can affect thinking. On the other hand, too much emphasis on the environment flies in the face of the clear evidence that human physiology is implicated in the evolution of depression. The days of looking for demons and spirits, chemicals and toxins, and bad parents and bad genes as single causative agents are past. None alone hold the key but collectively are a piece of the puzzle. This book attempts to describe depression, integrating the points of view of those who suffer from it, treat it, write about it, deal with it, legislate on it, and research it.

As a teacher, writer, clinician, citizen, and parent, I recognize my own different reactions to the broad topic of depression depending on my specific context. Integrating the reactions into one cohesive perspective was the challenge of the task at hand, that is, to write down the "life story of a disease," in this case, depression.

The subject matter of this book takes the reader on a journey of understanding depression from its descriptive past with romantic and spiritual narratives to a functional present with its physiological and technological explanations. Throughout the tome, the account of the experience of ordinary people shows time and again that a holistic conceptualization provides the best understanding to the illness of depression. To protect the identities of specific patients, I took their stories and clinical presentations and combined pertinent and illustrative facts into a composite account. I then created fictional patients and afflicted these imaginary characters with the composite symptoms.

My goal was to provide an airing of most of the major perspectives, without undue judgment or personal bias. My hope is that the curious high school student or college undergraduate reader will recognize the vastness of the topic and the myriad of possibilities and questions yet unanswered, and perhaps too have a deeper and more educated understanding when depression presents close to home.

ACKNOWLEDGMENTS

I want to recognize Lauren, Isabel, Anthony, Lucas, and Gabriel, who put up with my relative absence while writing this book and might have plunged into their own despair were it not for a great sense of humor and spirit of unselfish support. I also especially want to recognize my colleague and series editor Julie Silver, M.D., who was a tremendous cheerleader and source of encouragement throughout the process, and my editor, Kevin Downing at Greenwood, who put up with the many revisions and corrections, all the while displaying a tremendous sense of humor and sensibility. Finally, I want to thank Randy Baldini and Bob Seeley, both of whom were essential and supportive in the final edits.

Introduction

But when the melancholy fit shall fall
Sudden from heaven like a weeping cloud,
That fosters the droop-headed flowers all,
And hides the green hill in an April shroud.

from *Ode on Melancholy* (1819) by John Keats

This volume is one in a series of the biographies of diseases. They trace the histories of the diseases from the earliest recognition of their presence in humans through contemporary perspectives to imagining how the future will impact the way in which these conditions are considered.

The life in question here—the life of the clinical entity that is depression—is in many ways the most complicated of all the illnesses because, although it has been recognized for thousands of years and the descriptions of those afflicted today are similar to descriptions from 3,000 years ago, we still have very little fundamental understanding of how and why people get to depression, how best to treat it, or whether there is a possibility of a permanent cure. One reason for our lack of understanding is that depression affects the most complex of all the human organs, the brain. It is not simply the chemicals in the brain but the infinite ways in which brain nerves talk to each other in response to a person's environment, their genetics, and their very thinking that is implicated in depression. A brain paralyzed by depression is unable to begin to contemplate its own essence let alone the nature of any of the other disease states in this biographic series.

Before humans were able to communicate in a way that could be recorded, the prehistory of depression can only be inferred by extrapolating from the behavior of mammals whose evolutionary lines predated those of humans. The essential questions are as follows: How did it develop? What benefit did it offer our evolutionary forbears? And why does it persist today, especially if, in its most severe incantation, it kills those who suffer from it?

To contemplate these questions, the biography of the clinical condition of depression is explored using a genealogical approach, building incrementally through the ages on the wisdom of past thinkers. As with any family tree, there are dead ends comprising discredited theories and faulty treatment approaches, but these are essential in furthering our understanding. The truths that remain, those that are being tested now and those yet to be discovered, stand as a testament to our human desire to learn and our capacity to manipulate this knowledge so that perhaps one day Keats's "green hills" of vitality will no longer be hidden in the "April shroud" of depression.

1

What Is Depression?

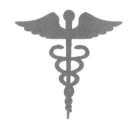

I am now the most miserable man living. If what I feel were equally distributed to the whole human family, there would not be one cheerful face on the earth. Whether I shall ever be better I cannot tell; I awfully forebode I shall not. To remain as I am is impossible; I must die or be better, it appears to me.

(Spiegel 2002, 199)

So wrote Abraham Lincoln on January 23, 1841, in a letter to John T. Stuart, his first law partner. Just what is it that drove Lincoln to write words laden with such despair? Lincoln shared a condition suffered by 20 million Americans today, and that is depression.

Depression is known clinically by various synonymous terms: major depressive disorder, major depression, clinical depression, or unipolar depression. The term unipolar is sometimes used because mood disorders are considered to be along a spectrum with two poles. One pole is depression, which is a low sad-feeling, mood state, and the other is mania, which is a high, elated, and agitated mood. People who suffer mood swings between these two poles are diagnosed as having bipolar illness. Bipolar depression refers to someone who has bipolar illness and is in his or her depressed state.

Although people afflicted by depression might express slightly different concerns, generally they describe having poor sleep and complain of low appetite, low energy, irritability, sadness, and loss of enjoyment in life. Sleep is a particularly troubling symptom. The sleep pattern can be one of either too much sleep or too little sleep and waking up frequently at night. In either case, the sleep is of poor quality, tormented by nightmares and provides little rest. A picture of such troubled sleep is described in Shakespeare's *Macbeth*, Act 2, Scene 1, in which Banquo says to Fleance:

> A heavy summons lies like lead upon me,
> And yet I would not sleep. Merciful powers,
> Restrain in me the cursèd thoughts that nature
> Gives way to in repose.

People with depression generally feel a loss of appetite, although others eat too much and then feel guilty about doing so and further feel worthless. They complain of a depressed mood, of losing interest in things in life that previously gave them pleasure, of feeling tired and fatigued. They can feel hopeless and helpless and guilty for all the bad things that happen in their lives and the world.

Author Elizabeth Wurtzel expressed her hopelessness less poetically but just as poignantly:

> I start to think there really is no cure for depression, that happiness is an ongoing battle, and I wonder if it isn't one I'll have to fight for as long as I live. I wonder if it's worth it.
>
> (Wurtzel 1995, 1)

Some will stop taking care of themselves and stop grooming, bathing, and taking care of other activities of daily living. People with depression can complain of physical symptoms such as headaches and stomachaches. The debilitation of depression can be so bad that they become overwhelmed with thoughts of suicide.

Chuck Palahniuk, the American novelist best known for his novel *Fight Club*, wrote about suicide thus:

> You have a choice. Live or die. Every breath is a choice. Every minute is a choice. To be or not to be.
>
> (Palahniuk 1999, 161)

Depression sufferers often feel profoundly alone. It is this loneliness that kills. In early 2007, Brad Delp, singer of the popular 1970s band Boston, committed suicide. He had written various notes. One in the garage read, "To whoever finds this I have hopefully committed suicide. Plan B was to asphyxiate myself in my car." A second note read, "I take complete and sole responsibility for my present situation. I have lost my desire to live." His suicide note read, "Mr. Brad Delp. J'ai une ame solitaire. I am a lonely soul."

Depression affects twice as many women as men. In a lifetime, depression will affect 10–25 percent of women and 5–12 percent of men. At any one point in time, 5–9 percent of women and 2–3 percent of men are likely to be clinically depressed. Some people have only one episode, but others have recurrent episodes of major depression. Some studies have shown that the more depressive episodes a person experiences, the less time there is between the episodes.

It is estimated that 10–25 percent of those who develop depression previously had dysthymia. Dysthymia—from the Greek *dys* (bad) and *thymia* (emotions)—is a disorder with similar but longer-lasting and milder symptoms than clinical depression. Generally, the symptoms must last two years to make the diagnosis, but the person is not as debilitated as someone with depression and is not suicidal.

Depression can also be associated with medical illnesses. Up to 20–25 percent of those who have illnesses such as cancer, stroke, diabetes, and myocardial infarction are likely to develop major depressive disorder sometime during the presence of their medical illness. Further depression can co-occur with other psychiatric illnesses, such as alcohol/drug abuse, anxiety disorders, obsessive-compulsive disorder, eating disorders, and borderline personality disorder.

Of all the statistics, none is more important than this: that up to 15 percent of people with major depression commit suicide. Sadly, many people who suffer from depression agree with Truman Capote:

> When you've got nowhere to turn, turn on the gas.
>
> (Capote 1987, 65)

The story of depression is one filled with drama, mystery, love, passion, and intrigue. It is a story told by ancient Greeks and presidents, prisoners and CIA agents, rock stars and ordinary citizens. It affects the young and the old, the rich and the poor, the Catholic and the Jew, the Black, the White, the Yellow, and the Brown. It is the story of evil spirits and abnormal chemicals, but universally it is a personal story impacting hope, life, and family, a story worth telling and worth knowing.

DEPRESSION DEFINED

> Depression is a prison where you are both the suffering prisoner and the cruel jailer.
>
> (Rowe 1983, 1)

The illness that plagued President Lincoln has captured the imagination of cartoonists and the curiosity of scientists. Depression has been defined by the wisdom of Charlie Brown and Eeyore, by the insights of poets, by entries in dictionaries, by clinicians in medical texts, and by the concern of advocacy groups.

The Clinicians

The American Psychiatric Association (APA) is a medical specialty society with more than 35,000 United States and international member physicians, mainly psychiatrists. It describes itself as "the voice and conscience of modern psychiatry," with a "vision as a society that has available, accessible quality psychiatric diagnosis and treatment."

The APA's major publication is the *Diagnostic and Statistical Manual of Mental Disorders* (DSM), which is a reference used by mental health professionals and physicians to diagnose mental disorders.

Although we will look at the criteria for depression more closely in Chapter 2, the DSM defines depression as a depressed mood state that lasts for at least two weeks and is accompanied by at least five of the following nine symptoms:

1. Feeling depressed, sad, blue, and tearful
2. Loss of interest or pleasure in things a person previously enjoyed doing
3. Increases or decreases in appetite and weight
4. Trouble sleeping or sleeping too much
5. Feeling either agitated or restless, or slowed down to an extent that others have begun to notice
6. Feeling tired or having no energy
7. Feelings of worthlessness or excessive guilt about things a person has done or not done
8. Trouble concentrating, thinking clearly, or making decisions
9. Feeling that they would be better off dead or having thoughts of suicide

The Cartoon Characters: Eeyore and Charlie Brown

Eeyore is the pessimistic, gloomy, depressed donkey and friend of Winnie-the-Pooh in the book series Winnie-the-Pooh by A. A. Milne. Eeyore can always be counted on to see the worst in every situation. For instance, in one scene, he is looking at his reflection in a stream:

"Pathetic," he said. "That's what it is. Pathetic." He turned and walked slowly down the stream for twenty yards, splashed across it, and walked slowly back on the other side. Then he looked at himself in the water again. "As I thought," he said. "No better from this side. But nobody minds. Nobody cares. Pathetic, that's what it is."

(Milne 1981, 72)

Eeyore's gloom is palpable, but he wasn't the only story character to suffer from depression. Made famous by cartoonist Charles Schulz, Charlie Brown is a child with endless determination and hope but who is nevertheless overwhelmed by depression, anxiety, and angst about the world. His perspective on depression is thus:

It always looks darkest just before it gets totally black.

(VanderHeyden 2003, 68)

He even had a way to stand when he was depressed:

This is my depressed stance. When you're depressed, it makes a lot of difference how you stand. The worst thing you can do is straighten up and hold your head high because then you'll start to feel better. If you're going to get any joy out of being depressed, you've got to stand like this.

Like these characters, real world poets, writers, and philosophers have attempted to capture the feeling of depression in words.

The Poets and Novelists

The Spanish philosopher George Santayana said:

Depression is rage spread thin.

(Applewhite, Frothingham, and Evans 1992, 50)

Judith Guest, the novelist best known for *Ordinary People*, had this perspective on depression:

Depression is not sobbing and crying and giving vent, it is plain and simple reduction of feeling.... People who keep stiff upper lips find that it's damn hard to smile.

(Guest 1976, 225)

The existential psychologist Rollo May was more succinct:

> Depression is the inability to construct a future.
>
> (Haas 1999, 74)

Perhaps it is best to end with William Styron, best-selling author of *Sophie's Choice* and his own memoir of living with depression, *Darkness Visible*:

> Depression is a disorder of mood, so mysteriously painful and elusive in the way it becomes known to the self—to the mediating intellect—as to verge close to being beyond description. It thus remains nearly incomprehensible to those who have not experienced it in its extreme mode.... The pain is unrelenting; one does not abandon, even briefly, one's bed of nails, but is attached to it wherever one goes.
>
> (Styron 1990, 7)

Although not as eloquent or pithy, more functional definitions of depression can be found in dictionaries.

The Dictionaries

In *The American Heritage Dictionary*, depression is defined as "a psychiatric disorder characterized by an inability to concentrate, insomnia, loss of appetite, anhedonia, feelings of extreme sadness, guilt, helplessness and hopelessness, and thoughts of death. Also called clinical depression."

In *Merriam-Webster's Medical Dictionary*, depression is "an act of depressing or a state of being depressed: as a (1) a state of feeling sad; (2) a psychoneurotic or psychotic disorder marked especially by sadness, inactivity, difficulty with thinking and concentration, a significant increase or decrease in appetite and time spent sleeping, feelings of dejection and hopelessness, and sometimes suicidal thoughts or an attempt to commit suicide."

The *Random House Unabridged Dictionary* defines depression as "a condition of general emotional dejection and withdrawal; sadness greater and more prolonged than that warranted by any objective reason."

The Government: The National Institutes of Mental Health

The National Institute of Mental Health (NIMH) is one of 27 components of the National Institutes of Health (NIH), the federal government's principal medical research agency. The NIH is part of the U.S. Department of Health and Human Services.

The NIMH states as its mission to "reduce the burden of mental illness and behavioral disorders through research on mind, brain, and behavior. This public health mandate demands that we harness powerful scientific tools to achieve better understanding, treatment, and eventually, prevention of these disabling conditions that affect millions of Americans."

The NIMH defines depression as follows: "A depressive disorder is an illness that involves the body, mood, and thoughts. It affects the way a person eats and sleeps, the way one feels about oneself, and the way one thinks about things. A depressive disorder is not the same as a passing blue mood. It is not a sign of personal weakness or a condition that can be willed or wished away. People with a depressive illness cannot merely 'pull themselves together' and get better. Without treatment, symptoms can last for weeks, months, or years. Appropriate treatment, however, can help most people who suffer from depression" (http://nimh.nih.gov).

The Nation's Largest Mental Health Advocacy Group: The National Alliance on Mental Illness

Founded in 1979, the National Alliance on Mental Illness (NAMI) is the nation's largest grassroots mental health organization dedicated to improving the lives of persons living with serious mental illness. The organization has become the nation's voice on mental illness, with chapters in every state and in more than 1,100 local communities, which join together to meet the NAMI mission through advocacy, research, support, and education.

Given NAMI's commitment to advocacy, their definition of depression is broad:

Major depression is a serious medical illness affecting 15 million American adults, or approximately 5 to 8 percent of the adult population in a given year. Unlike normal emotional experiences of sadness, loss, or passing mood states, major depression is persistent and can significantly interfere with an individual's thoughts, behavior, mood, activity, and physical health. Among all medical illnesses, major depression is the leading cause of disability in the United States and many other developed countries.

Depression occurs twice as frequently in women as in men, for reasons that are not fully understood. More than half of those who experience a single episode of depression will continue to have episodes that occur as frequently as once or even twice a year. Without treatment, the frequency of depressive illness as well as the severity of symptoms tends to increase over time. Left untreated, depression can lead to suicide.

Major depression, also known as clinical depression or unipolar depression, is only one type of depressive disorder. Other depressive disorders include dysthymia (chronic, less severe depression) and bipolar depression (the depressed phase of bipolar disorder or manic depression). People who have bipolar disorder experience both depression and mania. Mania involves unusually and persistently elevated mood or irritability, elevated self-esteem, and excessive energy, thoughts, and talking. (www.nami.org)

These definitions have helped modern-day sufferers recognize and identify a complex mental illness, the roots of which are buried deep in the very origins of humankind and are explored far more comprehensively in the next chapter.

ANCESTRAL DEPRESSION

In the Beginning

The creature, sensing the cold gloom of the day, walks into its cave to a far dark corner. Isolated, it will not eat or interact with others but crawls deep into the dark space and sleeps. Is this a form of depression? Perhaps, but it could just as easily describe hibernation, a state of inactivity and metabolic depression in animals, to conserve energy, especially during times of food scarcity. The body does what it does to protect itself.

Humans and their evolutionary ancestors have suffered from depression or an equivalent of depression ever since the nervous system became complex. There are many animal models of depression, and some prehistoric skulls have shown holes that were considered by anthropologists to have been drilled with the purpose of alleviating or dispelling evil spirits.

However, if depression, as with any other illness, were severe enough, it would compromise the species so much as to challenge the viability of the species. Yet depression exists in its various forms, so many evolutionary psychiatrists believe that depression has an evolutionary benefit.

One theory argues that depression benefits the animal in situations in which the ongoing effort to pursue something important will result in either danger or loss of resources. For instance, a fight with a dominant figure in the troupe to get a mate might lead to disaster, and so instead the animal shuts down and accepts its fate rather than lose life or limb.

As humans evolved, this adaptive function persisted. It would be useless for a person to continue to pursue a major goal and be consistently met with failure. The goal would not be achieved, and a tremendous amount of resources and energy that could have been deployed elsewhere and to the benefit of the family would be wasted. For this loss of energy not to occur, so that the person not continue to pursue his futile goal, an inhibitory response, including a reduction in energy, a slowing of the self, a loss of confidence and expectation, or hopelessness, would lead to a withdrawal from attempting the futile goal and thus ultimately conserve resources.

Furthermore, the evolutionary benefit of depression was not for the individual alone. Having a group of subordinate, less energetic more subdued individuals would ultimately preserve the stability of the whole social group, because having only highly competitive aggressive individuals would clearly not be a viable option.

It is also possible that what evolved was sadness and low energy states and that depression is simply a pathologic or more severe form of these states. It is also possible that different forms of depression evolved along different lines, and so our ancient and modern bear hibernating in the first paragraph could be a form or equivalent of seasonal affective disorder in humans.

All of this is theoretical and, although we can find ancient evidence of physical illness in the fossils of our ancestors, ancient evidence of depression, a mental condition, was not possible until humans found a way to communicate.

Although a written description of depression does not present until about 1500 BC, we do have evidence of the ancients attempting to treat the mind as long ago as 10,000 BC. Human skull fossils of the European Neolithic era have been found with what appear to be surgical holes in them. The process by which holes were drilled into the skulls of the afflicted is known as trephination.

Trephination was widely practiced by American Indians in Peru and Bolivia. Many of the trephined skulls show signs of healing after the holes were drilled, indicating that the patients survived after the operation, although some showed no such healing, indicating that the person died soon after the operation.

Although the particular afflictions for which trepanation was used are not known, the speculation is that it was used to either treat the wounds of battle or relieve the brain from the torment of the spirits that were believed to inhabit the brain.

The First Accounts

The archeological wealth of Egypt brought with it the discovery and translation of the so-called medical papyri, and it is clear that the ancient Egyptians took their health seriously.

The Ebers Papyrus dated about 1500 BC is probably the most important of the ancient medical papyri. Apart from containing prescriptions for about 700 remedies for various medical illnesses, it also contains a description of clinical depression with incantations and magic spells to be used to turn away the evil spirits that were thought to cause depression.

In Stanley Jackson's excellent book on the subject, *Melancholia and Depression: From Hippocratic Times to Modern Times*, he writes, "In ancient times, melancholia was attributed to 'black bile,' which was thought to wander around the body, finding no exit or escape. The treatment for the excess of this cold bile was purging, bloodletting, warm baths, exercise and proper diet" (Jackson 1986).

Hippocrates (ca. 460 BC to ca. 357 BC) was a Greek physician born in 460 BC on the island of Kos. He is known as the "father of medicine" because he based his practice on physical observations and on the study of the human body. He recognized that ill health had a physical explanation and was not caused by evil spirits, which was the prevailing theory of his day and parenthetically remains the belief in many cultures around the world today. His theory was that the body contained four bodily fluids or humors. The humors were phlegm, blood, black bile, and yellow bile. Illness came from a disturbance in the balance of any of the humors. The view of depression, or melancholia as it was known, was that there was an excess of black bile within the body. The word melancholia is a derivation of the Greek words for black (*melas*) and bile (*khole*).

The Greeks

Although healers of all types prevailed throughout the world, little is known of their practice for lack of any clear writings. The Greeks, who had

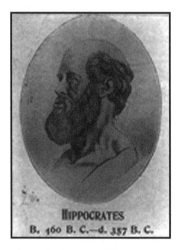

Figure 1.1. So powerful and convincing were Hippocrates' arguments that the concept that imbalances in the humors caused illness remained prevalent for the next 2,000 years. *Courtesy Library of Congress, Prints & Photographs Division, LC-USZ62-51385.*

produced Hippocrates, Plato, Aristotle, and countless other thinkers, artists, physicians, politicians, philosophers and so on, were careful archivists of their studies, and many of the writings remained or were cataloged by others.

After Hippocrates, Claudius Galen of Pergamum (130–200 AD) was arguably the next highly influential physician. He ultimately practiced in Rome and published more than 400 works on the practice of medicine! In his book *Functions of Diseases of Brain and Spinal Cord*, Galen wrote, "All of the best physicians and philosophers agree that the humors and actually the whole constitution of the body change the activity of the soul. If the first symptoms which appear in the stomach become more severe, they are followed by a melancholic affection. When a patient is relieved through bowel movements, vomiting, expulsion of flatus and belching, then we should rather call this illness hypochondriac and flatulent. If, however, the symptoms of melancholy become serious but the stomach is hardly involved then we should consider this disease as a primary affection of the brain due to an accumulation of black bile in this organ."

Because Galen believed that food was a primary cause of black bile, he cautioned against eating the meat of goats and oxen but that even worse was the meat of asses, camels, foxes, and dogs. Snails, wild boar, tuna, and dolphin were also cautioned against, as were the vegetables cabbage, brambles, and white rose. He also warned against drinking large quantities of red wine, especially in very hot climates, a caution that seems as relevant today as it was then.

The High Middle Ages

He who has white hair has a cold temperament; the hair of the warm temperament is black; he who is less cold will have tawny hair; he who is less warm will have reddish hair; the one with a balanced temperament has tawny hair mixed with red.

(Avicenna, from *The Poem on Medicine*)

After Galen, the medical world remained quiet on the subject of depression. Ibn Sina, known as Avicenna, was born in what is now modern-day Uzbekistan, of Persian origin, in 980 AD. He was a child prodigy who mastered algebra, philosophy, literature, and the Koran at a young age. He graduated in medicine at sixteen years of age. His great contribution to medicine was his massive four-volume *Canon of Medicine*, which was so influential that it was used as a medical reference for the next 600 years! It contained more than one million words. Gerard of Cremona translated it into Latin in the twelfth century, and his translation was widely read in Europe.

Like Hippocrates before him, Avicenna believed that melancholy was caused by a humoral imbalance. He postulated that melancholy (and all psychological problems) was caused by the overheating of black bile. By his description, symptoms of melancholy included flatulence, fears, and sleeplessness. Melancholic patients also had bad judgment, unreasonable fears, anger, loneliness, and tingling in the stomach. He also reported the curious symptom of patients having a craving for sex because of an excess of flatulence! A multitude of black body hair and body dryness were also sure signs, and, if this was not bad enough, nausea, feeling full and general stomach pains, followed by vomiting bile and sour food thereafter, completed the diagnosis.

The Renaissance

In the early Renaissance, Johan Weyer was the private physician of William, Duke of Cleves (who suffered from depression). The Duke protected Weyer and enabled him to speak out and reject the doctrine of witchcraft. Weyer said that natural causes of illness should be looked for in the mentally ill. As such, the physicians of the Renaissance believed that the ideas produced by the physicians of ancient Greece were correct and pertinent. Shakespeare's works are full of references to depression and the humors about which Galen had written.

During the Renaissance, the prominent French physician Andreas Laurentius (1558–1609) wrote, "there are four humours in our bodies, Blood, Phlegme, Choler and Melancholie; and that all these are to be found at all times in every age, and at all seasons to be mixed and mingled together within the veins, though not alike for everyone: for even as it is not possible to finde the partie in whom the foure elements are equally mixed ... there is alwaies someone which doth over rule the rest and of it is the partie's complexion named: if blood doe abound, we call such a complexion, sanguine; if phlegme, phlegmatic; if choler, cholerike; and if melancholie, melancholike."

Robert Burton

Robert Burton's *The Anatomy of Melancholy*, published in 1621, is arguably the first major text in the history of Western writing dedicated to mental illness. The original text was massive, containing more than 900 pages. In the book, he delves exhaustively into the causes of depression: "General causes are either supernatural or natural. Supernatural are from God and His angels, or by God's permission from the devil and his ministers."

Burton first cites biblical references showing God smiting his people with the likes of leprosy, dysentery, and other illnesses as punishment for various moral and other offenses, but it was not only the God of the monotheists who afflicted his people, but, as Burton puts it, the "heathen" gods similarly exacted revenge. Lycurgus, the King of Thrace, was driven to madness by Bacchus, the god of wine, for cutting down the vines in the country. Additional supernatural causes he considered were other nefarious spirits, fairies, satyrs and wood nymphs, ghosts, omens, witches, and magicians.

The other category of causes of depression were the natural causes. In this group, he included the stars, old age, parents, and bad diet. Although Burton was skeptical of the claims that the stars had much to do with melancholy, he noted that even Aristotle recognized that, after seventy years of age, it was clearly found in "weak and old persons," "especially such as have lived in action all their lives had great employment, much business, much command and many servants to oversee."

Burton seemed most convinced that a person's temperament, inherited from their parents, seemed a likely cause of depression. He considered these "inbred" causes. He wrote, "such as the temperature of the father is, such is the son's." As for the mother's contribution, he added, "If she be over-dull, heavy, angry, peevish, discontented, and melancholy, not only at the time of conception, but even all the while she carries the child in her womb, her son will be so likewise affected, and worse."

After considering the inbred methods, he moved onto the "outward and adventitious, which happen unto us after we are born." The outward causes were divided into the necessary (that is, those factors that were unavoidable) and the unnecessary.

The first of the outward causes he considered was diet and that it was the quality and quantity of "meat and drink" that caused melancholy by altering the humors of the body. Burton quoted Galen as saying that beef was particularly to blame. Pork was thought to be nutritious but not for those who were of unsound mind and body. Goat's flesh was thought to be particularly bad because it came from a "filthy beast." Essentially, Burton condemned all meat as possibly causing melancholy. As for milk he wrote, "milk and all that comes from milk increases melancholy." He recommended asses' milk as an exception to this consideration. He noted that milk was good for children for its nutritive quality except for when the milk had turned, or for children that had "unclean stomachs, are subject to headaches, or have green wounds."

He quoted physicians of the time who blamed fowl such as peacock and pigeons for causing melancholy and other physicians who felt that fish were slimy and of little nutritional value. Burton most strongly cautioned against spices, which cause melancholy, "to such men as are inclined to the malady."

Specifically, he mentioned pepper, ginger, cinnamon, cloves, and dates. Few foods appeared to be without their risk.

Although wine was considered to be risky by some, most physicians felt that, as he puts it, "a cup of wine is a good physic." Ciders were not advised because these were often spiced and therefore carried all the risks of the afore-mentioned spices. However, if the quality of the foods eaten were of concern, it was certainly the quantity that troubled Burton most. "Gluttony kills more than the sword," he wrote. "An insatiable paunch is the fountain of all diseases," he added.

The next group of outward causes was what he termed "retention and evacuation." These are essentially problems of constipation and other fluid retention. He presented a case thus: "A young merchant going to the Nordeling Fair in Germany, for ten days' space never went to stool; at his return he was grievously melancholy!" It was felt that the stool would back up the entire system and cause "inflammation in the head," leading to dulling of the senses and eventually melancholy. It probably remains true today that, whatever the cause, ten days of constipation would produce a seriously foul mood.

Other retention and evacuation problems included the presence of "hemrods (hemorrhoids), monthly issues in women and bleeding at nose." Yet another "retention" that was of serious concern to the physicians of the time was the lack of "venery" or the indulgence in or the pursuit of sexual activity. He quoted Pier Andrea Mattioli, an Italian physician, who wrote, "some through bashfulness abstained from venery and thereupon became heavy and dull." Again, the reason was that abstinence "sends up poisoned vapours to the brain and heart." Although physicians warned against abstinence for both men and women, they cautioned against "excessive venery." A patient was described thus: he married "a young wife and so dried himself with chamber-work, that he became in short space, from melancholy, mad." If too much or too little food and too much or too little sex were not enough to worry about, then the Renaissance man and woman had the quality of the air to consider, according to the French physician Fernel.

Jean François Fernel

Jean François Fernel described the cause of melancholy as "a thick air thickeneth the blood and humors." He warned against air that was too dry and hot and claimed that such air explained the high incidence of madness seen in Cyprus, Spain, and certain parts of Africa. The air around the other side of the equator was ideal, as evidenced, he suggested, by the "leaves ever green and cooling showers." The worst air, however, was "Thick, cloudy, misty foggy airs comes from moors where any carcasses lies, or from whence any stinking fulsome smell comes."

Aelianus Montaltus

Another perspective on the cause of depression was proposed by the physician Aelianus Montaltus who postulated that idleness was to blame: "They that are idle are far more subject to melancholy than such are conversant or employed about any office or business." Although idleness was considered a major cause of depression, exercising too much especially after eating meat led to corrupted undigested juices being taken into the veins and from there to the head.

An enforced solitariness, such as seen in monks, prisoners, and some students, was another cause of depression. Sleeping too much, which led to the brain being filled with nightmares, or too little and not allowing for enough rest were certain causes of melancholy.

Despite the various perspectives on the causes of depression, there were few novel perspectives on treatment. Those who thought that eating too much meat was the cause felt that eating less meat would be the cure. Those who felt that too much sleep led to the condition recommended sleeping less. In other words, the cure was reversing whatever excess was causing the depression. It was toward the end of the seventeenth century that a radical new treatment was considered.

Jean-Baptiste Denis and Richard Lower

The late 1600s brought with them the discovery of the circulation of blood by the physician William Harvey in England. This was soon followed by the first trial of transfusion of blood in animals. In 1666, an account of a successful transfusion in dogs was described in a letter by Dr. Richard Lower submitted to the Royal Society.

When reports of these experiments reached France, the Académie des Sciences immediately set about repeating them, and the first French experiments were the successful transfusion of blood between dogs. Dr. Denis took the experiments a step further when, in early 1667, he performed various experiments involving transfusion from three calves to three dogs. However, it was the transfusion of blood in humans that was of most interest to Denis and that ultimately led to his fame.

The first transfusion of blood in man was made on June 15, 1667, on a drowsy and feverish young man (Denis 1667). He received about twelve ounces of blood from a lamb, after which he "rapidly recovered from his lethargy, grew fatter and was an object of surprise and astonishment to all who knew him."

Richard Lower jumped on the transfusion bandwagon, and, in November 1667, Lower transfused Arthur Coga, "a mildly melancholy insane man," with the blood of a lamb. Coga described his experience in Latin before the Royal Society of Medicine and stated that he was much better. Depression had been treated by a blood transfusion!

After this, there was a short span of time when blood transfusions were taken as the cure for all ailments. Denis was most aggressive in these attempts and, in his second transfusion, gave the blood of a sheep to a forty-five-year-old chair bearer, who returned to work the next day as if nothing had happened to him. The third transfusion was on Baron Bonde, a young Swedish nobleman who fell ill in Paris while touring Europe. He was in such a bad state that he had been abandoned by his physicians and approached Denis requesting the new cure. After the first transfusion, which was from a calf, Bonde felt better and began to speak. This improvement lasted only a short time, however, and he died during a second transfusion.

A fourth transfusion patient was a paranoid man, Antoine Mauroy, who died during the procedure. Mauroy's wife accused Denis of having killed her husband. Denis brought the case before the court and he was cleared of any wrongdoing, but the court imposed the sanction that he could no longer perform the practice of transfusion of blood in humans without permission of the Paris Faculty of Medicine.

Further experiments inevitably led to the death of the recipient, and, as quickly as the practice of transfusions had become prominent, so it faded into obscurity.

From the early eighteenth century through the mid-nineteenth century, many of the mental hospitals that had appeared in early medieval times and had become prominent by the sixteenth and seventeenth centuries were reformed, changing them from dumping grounds for life's misfits to places were the mentally ill were humanely treated. Early reformers were Philippe Pinel in France, Vincenzo Chiarugi in Italy, and William Tuke in England, and millions of mentally ill patients owe their compassionate care to these three.

Philippe Pinel

Phillippe Pinel had originally set out to become a priest but later changed course and studied medicine. In 1789, he became a physician and wrote a book on the classification of diseases, which served as a standard medical textbook for schools of thought on clinical medicine. A defining moment in

Pinel's life was when a close friend of his became mentally ill and, during a severe psychotic break, ran into a forest and was devoured by a pack of wolves. Pinel moved from the practice of general medicine to devote his professional life to the care of the mentally ill. He began the practice of keeping case histories of all his patients, a practice that served as the basis for studying the course of mental illnesses.

In 1806, he published his *Treatise on Insanity*. In this work, he described a four-part diagnostic classification for the major mental illnesses: melancholy, dementia, mania without delirium, and mania with delirium. He also rejected the theory of humors as a form of ancient and medieval medicine. In the treatise, he wrote, "the symptoms generally comprehended by the term melancholia are taciturnity, a thoughtful pensive air, gloomy suspicions, and a love of solitude." He also noted that these characteristics however also described "some men in otherwise good health and frequently in prosperous circumstances." The distinction, he added, was the "brooding over his imaginary misfortunes."

He wrote that mental illness was caused by one or more of the following categories:

1. Harmful factors in the social environment such as a poor education
2. An irregular way of life
3. What he termed "spasmodic passions" in which he included rage and fright
4. Enervating or opposite passions (grief, hate, fear, remorse)
5. What he termed "the gay passions," meaning homosexual desire
6. A melancholic constitution
7. Physical factors such as alcoholism, hemorrhoids, child birth, and head injury
8. Heredity

The classification of mental illness developed by Pinel was an important contribution; however, more than this, it was his advocacy for the mentally ill that highlighted his career.

Increasingly, new ideas were proposed, each impacting the way depression was both considered and treated.

Franz Joseph Gall

One such idea was proposed by Franz Joseph Gall, who believed that specific brain areas controlled specific body functions and, furthermore, that character traits were related to the structure of certain areas within the brain. Gall's further assumption was that skull shape, particularly "bumps" on the skull, accurately reflected brain shape and therefore a person's character. The practice of character reading was developed and was known as "phrenology." It included the practice of measuring a person's skull. Most serious scientists paid little regard to the practice, but others used it as a way of "proving" the superiority and inferiority of different races.

Another concept was proposed by the surgeon Johann Christian Heinroth, who believed that a person's conflict between their acceptable impulses and their conscience was what caused mental illness. These ideas established the early thinking that would influence Freud to a significant extent.

Emil Kraepelin

In the last twenty years of the nineteenth century, German psychiatrist Emil Kraepelin introduced the first systematic classification of psychiatric disorders to be widely accepted. He identified the brain illness that later became known as schizophrenia. Ironically, while Freud was proposing psychological theories to explain mental illnesses, Kraepelin continued to assert their biological origin. Initially, he stated that these biological factors were primarily inherited but later shifted toward a belief in the importance of metabolic factors in mental illness.

The twentieth century brought an explosion in the understanding and treatment of depression. Research and statistics have made it easier for us to understand the extent and universality of the condition.

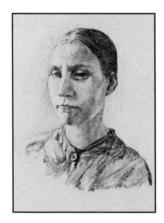

Figure 1.2. A late nineteenth-century portrait of a woman with melancholia. *Courtesy Library of Congress, Prints & Photographs Division, LC-USZ62-117381.*

THE EPIDEMIOLOGY OF DEPRESSION

Epidemiology is essentially the study of an illness, in this case depression. Epidemiological studies would therefore look at how many people have depression at a specific point in time and how many will go on to develop depression over their lifetime. It studies where those people are, how many new cases of depression develop, and how the depression is controlled. Epidemiological studies are generally done on many thousands of people to get the best possible picture of the problem. In the next chapter, we'll break down the big numbers to get more specific statistics such as the rates of depression in children and the elderly and the differences in men and women.

Because epidemiology measures illness not only at a specific point in time but in a specific location, rates of that illness can vary widely. Researchers have wondered whether this is true for major depression. Although epidemiology is mostly about statistics, these statistics are essential in helping health officials and lawmakers in deciding where and how to allocate resources.

Here is a look at the rates of depression as reported in various countries. This list is far from comprehensive but gives an indication of the epidemiology of depression across the globe.

United States

The Epidemiologic Catchment Area (ECA) program of research was initiated in response to the 1977 report of the President's Commission on Mental Health. The purpose was to collect data on the prevalence and incidence of mental disorders and on the use of and need for services by the mentally ill. In the research, more than 18,000 adults from five United States communities were interviewed. The research found that, at any given point in time, about 3 percent of all people were likely to be depressed. Another finding was that, over the course of a year, 9.5 percent of the U.S. population would suffer from some form of depression. In another nationwide survey, the National Comorbidity Survey, 8,098 people aged 15–54 years were assessed. Depression was found to be higher in women, young adults, and people with less than a college education. Furthermore, the chance of someone having an episode of depression at any point in their lifetime was about 17 percent.

Europe

Europe had their equivalent to the ECA, known as Outcomes of Depression International Network. The research looked at depression in the general population in five European countries and found that, similar to the United States, over the course of a year 8.56 percent of people would suffer from some form of depression, the rate being 10.05 percent for women and 6.61 percent for men. The rate was highest in urban Ireland and urban United Kingdom and lowest in urban Spain. In another study, a randomized telephone survey of 18,980 subjects aged fifteen years and older among the general populations of the United Kingdom, Germany, Italy, Portugal, and Spain, depression at that any given point in time was found to be 4 percent (3.1 percent in men and 4.9 percent in women), which again, is similar to U.S. statistics.

Finland

Although Finland is part of the European Union, it has anecdotally been considered to have higher rates of depression than the rest of the union. The thinking is that, due to the long winter months with very little sunshine, the Finnish population is at greater risk for depression. They are considered to be a very reserved people, even by the Finns themselves. Merete Mazzarella, a professor of Nordic literature at the University of Helsinki, tells a joke: "How do you know if the Finn on the elevator with you is outgoing? When he's looking at your shoes instead of at his own."

Some researchers view the Finnish reticence as more pathological, linking it to depression, citing the Finns' high rates of suicide and alcoholism. This reticence pervades Finnish society. Eeyore (Milne's character) would have agreed with this perspective from psychologist Liisa Keltikangas-Järvinen, at the University of Helsinki. "In Swedish they say 'great" all the time. In Finnish we don't say that things are great. We just don't. Things are OK or maybe good." She goes on to say that children are taught early on to resist their impulses and that boasting about personal accomplishments is the worst thing a Finn can do. "If you can't control yourself, you are regarded as immature," she added.

Given these concerns, epidemiologists looked at the rates of depression in Finland. In the Mini-Finland Health Survey (Lehtinen et al. 1990), which comprised a total of 8,000 persons representing the whole adult population of Finland (aged thirty years or more), depression at any point in time was 3.6 percent in men and 5.5 percent in women. Another research study (Lindeman et al. 2000) reported on the rate of depression occurring over the course of a year and found 9.3 percent of Finns were likely to suffer from a depressive episode, with the rate for females being 10.9 percent and for males 7.2 percent.

These figures are not all that different from those for the United States or the rest of Europe, so despite their reputation the Finns are in fact not more depressed than the rest of their northern hemisphere peers.

Saudi Arabia

It is often the case that there are fewer epidemiologic research studies in poorer nations than richer ones specifically because of lack of resources. Interestingly, there is less research into depression in Saudi Arabia than might be expected from this cash- and resource-rich country. One large study on depression in the elderly population of Saudi Arabia with nearly 8,000 participants averaging sixty-nine years of age found that depressive symptoms were reported in 39 percent of the subjects.

Another small study among adolescents found that more than 20 percent of adolescents were depressed, with adolescent girls in Saudi Arabia being 1.5 times more likely to suffer from depression than adolescent males.

Cross-National Studies

Some researchers have taken on the mammoth task of collaborating with colleagues from around the world to obtain statistics from across the globe at a similar point in time. One study (Weissman et al. 1996) researched the rates of depression in 38,000 people in ten countries: the United States, Canada, Puerto Rico, France, West Germany, Italy, Lebanon, Taiwan, Korea, and New Zealand. The researchers found that the rate of developing depression at any point in their lifetime varied widely across countries, ranging from 1.5 cases per 100 adults in the sample from Taiwan to 19.0 cases per 100 adults in Beirut.

At any given point in time, the rate of depression varied from a low of 0.8 cases per 100 adults in Taiwan to 5.8 cases per 100 adults in New Zealand. In every country, the rates of major depression were higher for women than men.

In their study, the researchers found that poor sleep and loss of energy occurred in most people with major depression in each country. Also, they found that people with major depression were also at increased risk to suffer from substance abuse and anxiety disorders. People who were separated or divorced had significantly higher rates of major depression than married people, and the risk was somewhat greater for divorced or separated men than women.

The Bottom Line

Whether national agencies, well-funded university research, or less-well-funded individual researchers conduct studies, there appear to be marked similarities in the rates of depression across countries. In all countries, clinical depression is a major healthcare problem that requires ongoing focus and research.

The statistics of epidemiology are dry and impersonal; they are, however, the essential tools for increasing awareness to the magnitude of a problem, in this case depression. A much more passionate approach to increasing public and political awareness of the suffering of depression is the creative output of artists and poets, an approach that we will review in the next section.

DEPRESSION IN THE ARTS

> Melancholy is not *only* negative. On the contrary, it was a positive energy that gave strength and genius to great artists throughout Western civilization.
>
> (Gérard Régnier, director of the Musée Picasso in Paris)

The relationship between art and the mental condition of melancholia or depression has existed for as long as humans were able to express themselves in all forms of artistic endeavor. The ancient Greeks believed in divine forms of madness that inspired mortals' creative acts or performances. In her book *Touched with Fire: Manic-Depressive Illness and the Artistic Temperament*, Kay Redfield Jamison wrote, "To assume that such diseases usually promote artistic talent wrongly reinforces simplistic notions of the 'mad genius.' ... All the same, recent studies indicate that a high number of established artists meet the diagnostic criteria for depression.... In fact, it seems that these diseases can sometimes enhance or otherwise contribute to creativity." (Jamison 1995, 62–67). Psychiatrist Arnold Ludwig, in his book *The Price of Greatness: Resolving the Creativity and Madness Controversy*, has looked at the statistics (Ludwig 1995). He spent ten years looking at the lives of 1,004 deceased men and women who had lived during the twentieth century and gained prominence in the arts and other fields such as the sciences, public office, and business. He found that about one-third of the eminent poets, musical performers, and fiction writers suffered from serious psychological symptoms of some kind as teenagers and that this number had increased to about three-quarters by the time they reached adulthood! Of particular note was that 46–77 percent of poets, fiction and nonfiction writers, painters, and composers encountered periods of serious depression, more than twice the rate observed in people in other professional fields.

Whether this is cause or effect is harder to tease out. Some endeavors, such as painting, poetry, and fiction writing, more readily tolerate ambiguity and flexibility in expression, and so it seems clear that these fields will more readily accept practitioners with mental disorders as they struggle with their inner turmoil. Professions that emphasize structure and predictability, such as science, tend to attract and promote people with less disorganization. The creative output for artists is often its own reward, and some endure the lows of depression for the moments of joy. The author Agatha Christie wrote, "I like living. I have sometimes been wildly, despairingly, acutely miserable, racked with sorrow, but through it all I still know that just to be alive is a grand thing" (Goldsmith 2002, 228).

Fine art, poetry, literature, music, theater, and film have all tackled the subject of depression. Many artists and producers were themselves influenced by depression during their creative efforts. Depression was not typically considered an obstacle to creativity but rather a force that led to artistic innovation by stimulating an intensity of emotion, which in turn fostered the artist's creative powers. Over time, however, an artist's depression became less the muse or inspiration than the debilitating illness that it is. Ernest Hemingway in a letter to F. Scott Fitzgerald (Mellow 1993, 390) wrote, "That terrible mood of depression of whether it's any good or not is what is known as The Artist's Reward." Hemingway, burdened by crippling depression, attempted suicide in the spring of 1961 and received electroconvulsive therapy (ECT) treatment. On July 2, 1961, at his home in Idaho, he killed himself with a shotgun blast to the head. His father, bother, sister, and actress daughter Margaux all suffered from depression and also committed suicide. Whether a creativity inspiring influence, a life-destroying illness, or both, depression has been captured in the art of many. Some examples follow.

Poetry

Nicholas Breton

Above, we saw Robert Burton become a celebrity with his wordy publication *The Anatomy of Melancholy* in 1621. Elizabethan England seemed both riddled with and obsessed by depression, and there was much literature dedicated to the matter. An early example of depression in poetry is the poem *A Briefe of Sorrowe*, published in 1600 by Nicholas Breton:

Muse of sadness, neere deaths fashion,
Too neere madnesse, write my passion.
Paines possesse mee, sorrows spill me,
Cares distress me, all would kill mee.
Hopes have faild me, Fortune foild mee,
Feares have quaild me, all have spoild mee.
Woes have worne mee, sighes have soakt mee,
Thoughts have torne mee, all have broke mee.

Beauty strooke me, love hath catcht mee,
Death hath tooke mee, all dispatcht mee.

Depression inspired not only the Elizabethan poets but also those who followed.

William Cowper

Cowper was an English poet and hymnodist. He suffered from periods of severe depression and turned to Christianity for comfort. Despite this, he experienced at least four crippling bouts of clinical depression and he feared that he was doomed to eternal damnation. In 1752, he sank into his first paralyzing depression, and he wrote about this episode thus:

> [I was struck] with such a dejection of spirits, as none but they who have felt the same, can have the least conception of. Day and night I was upon the rack, lying down in horror, and rising up in despair. I presently lost all relish for those studies, to which before I had been closely attached; the classics had no longer any charms for me; I had need of something more salutary than amusement, but I had not one to direct me where to find it.
>
> (Hayley 1851, 508)

More than thirty years later, he shared his reflections in a letter to his close friend John Newton. He wrote:

> Loaded as my life is with despair, I have no such comfort as would result from a supposed probability of better things to come, were it once ended.... You will tell me that this cold gloom will be succeeded by a cheerful spring, and endeavour to encourage me to hope for a spiritual change resembling it—but it will be lost labour. Nature revives again; but a soul once slain lives no more.... My friends, I now expect that I shall see yet again. They think it necessary to the existence of divine truth, that he who once had possession of it should never finally lose it. I admit the solidity of this reasoning in every case but my own. And why not in my own? ... I forestall the answer:—God's ways are mysterious, and He giveth no account of His matters:—an answer that would serve my purpose as well as theirs that use it. There is a mystery in my destruction, and in time it shall be explained.
>
> (Thomas 1935, 281–282)

John Keats

In the spring of 1819, John Keats, one of the principal poets of the English Romantic movement, wrote the following in a letter to his brother George and sister Fanny:

> Circumstances are like Clouds continually gathering and bursting— while we are laughing the seed of some trouble is put into the wide arable land of events—while we are laughing it sprouts it grows and suddenly bears a poison fruit which we must pluck.
>
> (Motion 1999, 22)

Keats struggled with depression during the latter part of his life. His depression was made all the worse by his wife leaving him and the harsh critique of his work by the London literature critics. He was inspired to write his *Ode on Melancholy* (1819). In it, he recognized that joy and pain were inseparably linked and that, to experience joy fully, we had to experience depression fully:

> Ay, in the very temple of delight
> Veil'd Melancholy has her Sovran shrine,
> Though seen of none save him whose strenuous tongue
> Can burst Joy's grape against his palate fine;
> His soul shall taste the sadness of her might,
> And be among her cloudy trophies hung.

Jean-Jacques Rousseau and Lord Byron

Jean-Jacques Rousseau was a Genevan philosopher whose political ideas influenced the French Revolution. He was instrumental in the development of socialist theory and made important contributions to literature and music as both a theorist and a composer. As with many innovators of his time, his ideas were not well accepted by everyone and he encountered significant persecution, which lead to a serious decline in his mental health and ultimately a crippling psychotic depression. The nineteenth-century poet Lord Byron himself endured what he called "savage moods." He had a creative spirit similar to Rousseau's, whose writings made a deep impression on the poet's mind. Of Rousseau, Byron wrote the following:

> Here the self-torturing sophist, wild Rousseau,
> The apostle of affliction, he who threw
> Enchantment over passion, and from woe

Wrung overwhelming eloquence, first drew
The breath which made him wretched; yet he knew
How to make madness beautiful. . . .

(Goode 1972, 233)

Books

As in poetry, the suffering of men and women afflicted by depression has inspired many books. Some accounts were fictional and others biographical. Of the fictional greats who struggled with depression, few are better known than Shakespeare's Hamlet whose symptoms practically define depression. Some scholars have argued that Shakespeare's descriptions were so accurate that he must have suffered from depression himself.

William Shakespeare

In *Hamlet*, Act 1, Scene 2, Shakespeare writes:

O God, God,
How weary, stale, flat, and unprofitable
Seem to me all the uses of this world?
Fie on't, ah fie, 'tis an unweeded garden
That grows to seed. Things rank and gross in nature
Possess it merely.

Again quoting from *Hamlet*, Shakespeare writes this about suicidal thinking:

O that this too too sullied flesh would melt
Thaw, and resolve itself into a dew,
Or that the Everlasting had not fixed
His canon 'gainst self-slaughter.

Then in Act 2, Scene 2, Shakespeare writes the following on the loss of interest in pleasure:

I have of late, but wherefore I know not, lost all my mirth, forgone all custom of exercise; and indeed, it goes so heavily with my disposition that this goodly frame, the earth, seems to me a sterile promontory; this most excellent canopy, the air, look you, this brave o'erhanging firmament, this majestical roof fretted with golden fire: why, it appears no other thing to me than a foul and pestilent congregation of vapours.

Shakespearian scholars have hypothesized that Shakespeare must have suffered from depression. The two major arguments are that he wrote so clearly on the subject and that his writing starting with and after *Hamlet* was filled with melancholy, death, and dread and not the mirth and playfulness of his earlier works, but Shakespeare left no autobiographical material that helps to clearly answer the question. Today's authors address the subject directly, many describing their own personal experience.

Johann Wolfgang Goethe

Johann Wolfgang Goethe was a late eighteenth-century German poet, novelist, dramatist, theorist, painter, natural scientist, and government minister. He was a prolific writer who also suffered from crippling bouts of depression. One of his most famous literary works is *The Sorrows of Young Werther* published in 1774. The novel is considered to be autobiographical given the unquestionable parallels between Goethe and the book's main character Werther. In 1772, when Goethe was an unknown legal apprentice, he fell desperately in love with Charlotte Buff. Buff was engaged to his close friend Kestner. Unable to have Buff, Goethe fell into a severe depression and considered suicide. In the book, Goethe tells the story of young Werther who suffers the extremes of unrequited love and eventually commits suicide. The book became an instant bestseller, and "Werther fever" consumed Germany. Clusters of suicides occurred in young German men who dressed up in Werther's yellow waistcoat and blue coat and then, like Werther, shot themselves. Goethe himself chose to suffer with his depression and died of natural causes at eighty-two years of age.

Andrew Solomon

Andrew Solomon, from his autobiographical *The Noonday Demon: An Atlas of Depression,* has been insightfully articulate on the condition: "Depression is the flaw in love. To be creatures who love, we must be creatures who can despair at what we lose, and depression is the mechanism of that despair. When it comes, it degrades one's self and ultimately eclipses the capacity to give or receive affection. It is the aloneness within us made manifest, and it destroys not only connection to others but also the ability to be peacefully alone with oneself" (Solomon 2001, 15). Solomon recognized that he felt that his depression started with the traumatic death of his mother. Following her death, he described feeling a "creeping numbness" that made him stop caring about what was happening to him. After the numbness, he felt overwhelmed by the simplest of tasks. He describes the act of preparing a meal, thus: "The idea that in order to eat, one has to get the food out of the fridge and put it on a plate, and cut it up and lift it to one's mouth and chew it and swallow it—it seemed so difficult to me, I wondered how someone else was able to get through it."

Kay Redfield Jamison

Kay Redfield Jamison is a psychologist and professor of psychiatry at the Johns Hopkins University School of Medicine. She has written extensively on the subject of mental illness and, in particular, bipolar depression, including her own memoir *An Unquiet Mind: A Memoir of Moods and Madness*. In describing just how incapacitating her depression was, she said, "Depressed, I have crawled on my hands and knees in order to get across a room and have done it for month after month" (Jamison 1997). More than a writer on the subject, she is an advocate for better mental healthcare. In *Night Falls Fast: Understanding Suicide*, she wrote: "Every seventeen minutes in America, someone commits suicide.... Mostly, I have been impressed by how little value our society puts on saving the lives of those who are in such despair as to want to end them. It is a societal illusion that suicide is rare. It is not" (Jamison 2001, 299).

William Styron

Another brilliant writer on the subject of depression is William Styron, probably most famous for his novel *Sophie's Choice*. Like the aforementioned authors, he had the genes and circumstances that predisposed him to depression. His childhood was a difficult one, with his father also suffering from clinical depression and his mother dying of cancer before his fourteenth birthday. In *Darkness Visible: A Memoir of Madness*, he speaks about resilience and recovery from depression: "One need not sound a false or inspirational note to stress the truth that depression is not the soul's annihilation; men and women who have recovered from the disease—and they are countless—bear witness to what is probably its only saving grace: it is conquerable" (Styron 1990, 84).

Brooke Shields

Another account is that of actress Brooke Shields in her autobiography *Down Came the Rain: My Journey Through Postpartum Depression*. Nothing should have made her happier than becoming pregnant. She had completed several series of in vitro fertilization treatments and had a painful miscarriage. After many attempts, she became pregnant. After the birth of her daughter Rowan, something went terribly wrong as she slipped into depression. She describes the beginning of the struggle thus: "I started to experience a sick sensation in my stomach; it was as if a vise was tightening around my chest. Instead of the nervous anxiety that often accompanies panic, a feeling of quiet devastation overcame me. I hardly moved. Sitting on my bed, I let out a deep, slow, guttural wail. I wasn't simply emotional or weepy like I had been told I might be. This was something quite different" (Shields 2005, 65).

Music

I have suffered from depression for most of my life. It is an illness.
                                        (Adam Ant, 1980s British rock star)

Each artist chooses his or her medium for expression, and the expression of depression in the lyrics of contemporary music can be as clear as that of the spoken or written word.

Van Morrison

In 1997, Irish rock star Van Morrison gave an interview to Entertainment Weekly in which he admitted that he suffered from depression: "People get depressed. It's a fact of life. So, write a song about that. Write a song about melancholia, which is just the blues, anyway, under a different name" (Gordinier 1997).

He had done just that when he wrote the song "Underlying Depression" from the 1995 collection *Days Like This*. Familiar themes of depression are reflected in the lyrics "Underlying depression, have to crawl into my room," noting withdrawal and isolation, and "Underlying depression and there's just nowhere to turn," speaking to the hopelessness of depression. The song is not all loss of hope as he battles on, with a vow to fight with all that it takes, recognizing that in fact he has plenty for which to be grateful.

James Taylor

Another music great who suffered from depression was James Taylor. As a teen, he was hospitalized at McLean Hospital in Belmont, Massachusetts. This was a time that inspired many of his early songs. His struggles with depression and drug addiction have been well chronicled. Like Morrison, Taylor too wrote a song about his struggle with depression in "Another Grey Morning." His experience resonates as he sings of the greyness of his days and that "no one seems to care." As he spirals into the hopelessness of his situation, he concludes his song with the contemplation of most who suffer with depression: "But no more grey morning. I think I'd rather die." Taylor eventually overcame his depression and thoughts of death to become one of the most prolific singer/song writers ever.

Theater

Theater has tackled depression as a subject matter but faces the difficult challenge of keeping the audience interested without letting the morbidity of the theme in turn depress its watchers. Because of this, many plays on depression infuse a thread of humor in their story.

The Disappearance of Janey Jones is a play by Jennifer Fawcett and tells the story of the mind of Janey Jones as she slips into depression. She considers her lot as she lies in bed after her grandmother has just committed suicide, and it is the morning of her funeral. To make matters worse, she's lost her job, she's lost her relationship, and she's starting to think she may be following the same path as her grandmother. The history of Janey's depression unfolds as she is visited by characters from her past, her mother, her childhood self, and her psychiatrist, often with comedic effect.

A different approach is *The Depression Show* by Thomas Keith and Jane Young, in which four depressed people endure the inquisition of a ridiculously happy television talk-show host and hostess who grin their way through the interview of their guests into revealing their illnesses on camera. A psychoanalyst reassures the hapless four that they will all be fine. The show is less about making fun of the depressed than of television talk shows, a public that will watch anything, and cheerleading psychologists.

Finally, *How to Fake Clinical Depression* by Steven Marrocco tells the story of a broke and destitute actor who decides to make some money by taking part in a study testing a new antidepressant medication. A major drug company is offering $1,000 to depressed people to participate in their study. He trains himself to fake a depression to be allowed into the study, and, in the process, experiences the highs and lows that come with his choices, learns a little about happiness.

Film

It is impossible these days to walk through a checkout aisle and not see the many faces of mental illness plastered on the celebrity magazines. Drug abuse, alcoholism, anorexia, the consequences of divorce, rage, violence, and abuse are on display for the world to see. The actors and actresses of Hollywood have their real-life mental torment exposed to an insatiable public as readily as Hollywood likes to make fictional accounts of these conditions.

The Academy of Motion Picture and Arts frequently awards its Oscars to characters with serious mental problems. *A Beautiful Mind* won the Oscar for Best Movie in 1991 with Russell Crowe portraying schizophrenia. In 1996, the Oscar winning film was *The English Patient* in which Ralph Fiennes depicts a man with amnesia and flashbacks. The 1994 winner *Forrest Gump* has Tom Hanks as a mental simpleton with all the answers. In 1991, Anthony Hopkins is a psychopathic cannibal in *The Silence of the Lambs*. In 1997, Jack Nicholson won the Best Actor Oscar for his role as a man suffering from obsessive-compulsive disorder in *As Good as it Gets* (and, incidentally, he won an Oscar in 1975 for his role as a mental patient in *One Flew Over the Cuckoos Nest*). Charlize Theron won the Best Actress Oscar in 2003 as a demented serial killer in *Monster*, and Nicole Kidman won hers in 2003 playing the role of the depressed Virginia Woolf in *The Hours*. The list is near endless and perhaps provides a formula for Oscar success. Two movies that look at depression specifically are below.

The Hours (2003)

The Hours takes place over three periods of time and focuses on the lives of three women, all of whom suffer from depression. It portrays the hopelessness of depression and the viability of the option of suicide as a solution to depression and depicts the various reactions that a person's depression has on the people who love them. The first woman is the English author Virginia Woolf (played by Nicole Kidman) who, in 1923, is trying to write her latest novel, *Mrs. Dalloway*. She had moved from London to Richmond with her husband because he hoped that the move would help her get over her clinical depression. In the movie, Woolf plans a party hoping that a visit from her sister will cure her of her intense depression. Neither the move nor the visit lift Woolf's depression, and she ultimately commits suicide by drowning.

Next is Laura Brown (played by Julianne Moore) living in Los Angeles in 1951. She is a depressed housewife with a loving and supportive husband and her young son, who also loves her. She is pregnant with her second child but feels miserable despite her loving family. The very act of baking a birthday cake for her husband makes her feel suicidal. All the wonderful things in her life are not enough to lift her depression, but she happens to be reading *Mrs. Dalloway*, which gives Laura insight into her own torment and so she decides not to kill herself.

Finally, there is Clarissa Vaughan (played by Meryl Streep) who plays a lesbian book editor in New York City in 2001. She is busy planning a party for her former lover Richard, a gay man who is in the last stages of AIDS. His pet name for her is "Mrs. Dalloway" because the character in Virginia Woolf's book is named Clarissa and she shares the character's need to throw parties and look after others, but Clarissa is not herself happy. Neither Clarissa's partner Sally, nor her daughter, nor her friends understand why she is depressed, and, in the planning of the party, she is jolted into the awareness that her own life, her own happiness, and her own needs have taken a back seat to taking care of Richard.

A more contemporary look at depression in film, one that deals with issues of therapy, medication, prescribing practices, overmedication, suicide, and environmental factors that contribute to depression, is *Garden State*.

Garden State (2004)

In *Garden State*, Andrew (played by Zach Braff) suffers from depression, for which he has been highly medicated since the age of nine. His psychiatrist father has prescribed all his medications, and there are scenes of his medicine cabinet well stocked with bottles of various antidepressants. Sadly, this portrayal of the medication cabinet of a person suffering from depression is not hyperbole, because all too often patients have been tried on multiple trials of medication before "something works." Dangerously, the old medication bottles are often left partially full in the medication cabinets, and, in rare instances, a cocktail of these unused medications is consumed in a suicide attempt.

In the movie, his current medications appear to quell his depression, but, as is true of the treatment of depression, medications do not address the events in a person's life that underlie the depression. For instance, he feels responsible for the paralysis of his mother who was injured in an accident. In the movie, he returns to New Jersey for his mother's funeral and he decides to stop taking his medication because he wants to get out of his pill-induced funk. People with depression often complain of a sense of being "chemically" normal or happy and often advocate strongly with their psychiatrists that they want to stop taking the medication. At times, when psychiatrists recommend against such a move, patients will precipitously take themselves off medications, which can lead to serious side effects.

Having defined depression, looked at how the ancients thought of the condition, identified who suffers from it today, and seen how people have artistically portrayed or been influenced by the illness, we move away from a more narrative, descriptive perspective to a more scientific, data-driven view of depression.

2

How Is Depression Diagnosed?

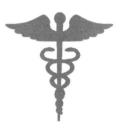

Our understanding of depression has come a long way since the ancient Greeks worked their medicine trying to correct the humoral imbalances that they were convinced caused the illness. Here we look at a more contemporary understanding of the condition.

MAKING THE DIAGNOSIS OF DEPRESSION

Psychiatrists use the *Diagnostic and Statistical Manual of Mental Disorders* (DSM) to make psychiatric diagnoses. The criteria from the DSM for a major depressive episode are listed below. To be diagnosed with depression, a person must have at least five of the following nine symptoms, which must have been present during the same two-week period of time.

1. The first is a depressed mood most of the day, nearly every day, as indicated by either subjective report (the person feels sad or empty) or the observation made by others (that the person appears tearful). For people suffering from depression, the dread of the depressed mood feels as if it will never end. Author Elizabeth Wurtzel wrote, "That's the thing about depression: A human being can survive almost

anything, as long as she sees the end in sight. But depression is so insidious, and it compounds daily, that it's impossible to ever see the end. The fog is like a cage without a key." In Psalms 6:2, a depressed King David laments, "How long shall I take counsel in my soul, having sorrow in my heart daily? How long shall mine enemy be exalted over me?"

2. There is a markedly diminished interest or pleasure in all, or almost all, activities most of the day, nearly every day. F. Scott Fitzgerald said, "Every act of life, from the morning toothbrush to the friend at dinner, became an effort. I hated the night when I couldn't sleep and I hated the day because it went toward night" (Oates 2001, 142).

3. There is significant weight loss when not dieting or weight gain (e.g., a change of more than 5 percent of body weight in a month) or decrease or increase in appetite nearly every day.

4. Another symptom is insomnia (which is an inability to sleep) or hypersomnia (far too much sleep) nearly every day. Generally, people with depression complain of an inability to sleep, when they simply lie in bed tormented by thoughts of how terrible they feel. "Insomnia is a gross feeder. It will nourish itself on any kind of thinking, including thinking about not thinking," so wrote author Clifton Fadiman. As F. Scott Fitzgerald put it, "The worst thing in the world is to try to sleep and not to."

5. There is psychomotor agitation or retardation nearly every day. This means that the person appears or feels slowed down.

6. There is fatigue or loss of energy nearly every day. "Our fatigue is often caused not by work, but by worry, frustration and resentment," said Dale Carnegie (2004, 219). The draining effects of depression are far more burdensome and fatigue inducing than those of physical activity.

7. The person complains of feelings of worthlessness or excessive or inappropriate guilt (which may be delusional) nearly every day. This guilt can at times be delusional because the things that a person feels they have done are often not as bad as their loved ones or objective observers would consider. Nevertheless, guilt can powerfully color depression a darker shade of black. The American Theologian noted that "Guilt is the very nerve of sorrow," a sentiment that resonates with many who suffer from depression.

8. The person has diminished ability to think or concentrate, or is indecisive, nearly every day.

9. There are recurrent thoughts of death, with or without a plan, or a suicide attempt. The symptoms cause clinically significant distress or

impairment in social, occupational, or other important areas of functioning. Joseph Conrad said, "Suicide, I suspect, is very often the outcome of mere mental weariness not an act of savage energy but the
final symptom of complete collapse." Once again, King David in
Psalms 13:4 said, "My heart is sore pained within me: and the terrors
of death are fallen upon me."

TYPES OF DEPRESSION

Other than major depression and dysthymia, there are other forms or variations of depression recognized by mental health professionals.

Postpartum depression is a form of major depression suffered by about
10 percent of new mothers. It is more common in women who have already suffered from some form of depressive illness. Perhaps one of the most talked about
cases of postpartum depression was that of Brooke Shields, who wrote about her
experience with the condition after the birth of her daughter. Many cannot
imagine how someone who seemingly has it all, beauty, wealth, fame, and a
seemingly happy marriage, could possibly be depressed, especially after the birth
of a child. Yet, after her child was born, she struggled with a crippling bout of
postpartum depression. She stated, "I really didn't want to live anymore. 'I just
want to leap out of my life,' but then the rational side of me says 'you're only
on the fourth floor. You'll get broken to bits and then you will be even worse.'"

There is atypical depression, which usually begins in adolescence and is
more commonly seen in women. Symptoms such as oversleeping, overeating,
and being extremely sensitive to rejection are characteristic of atypical depression. It is called atypical because, although there is a depressed mood, "typical" symptoms such as insomnia and low appetite are not present.

Premenstrual dysphoric disorder is a condition experienced by about
5 percent of menstruating women. It is different from premenstrual syndrome
in that the symptoms of depression are more severe and last longer, and it is
associated with more irritability.

Psychotic depression is a type of depression in which the person begins to
imagine or hear and see things that have no basis in reality. I remember as a
young resident in psychiatry a patient told me "Beginning about three years
ago, I began to have regular bouts of depression that would happen every two
to three months. They would last a couple of weeks. At first, the depression
was just a low mood, and I blamed myself for feeling that way. But as the episodes became more severe, I had frightening hallucinations; I started hearing
voices, seeing distorted faces, demons, and the devil, and thought that they
were out to take me to hell."

Then there is bipolar depression, which is the low mood phase of manic-depressive illness. It is important to make the distinction between major depression and bipolar depression because treating a patient with bipolar depression with an antidepressant alone can cause the person to become manic, which is the up phase of the condition. Both phases of the condition can disrupt a life. Kay Redfield Jamison described it thus: "Depressed, I have crawled on my hands and knees in order to get across a room and have done it for month after month. But normal or manic I have run faster, thought faster, and loved faster than most I know."

Seasonal depression or seasonal affective disorder is a type of depression whose symptoms are recognized as worsening during changes in season. Generally, people who suffer from this form of depression are especially sensitive to the diminishing hours of daylight in the late fall or early winter. I recently saw a twenty-five-year-old school teacher who presented one October complaining of increasing fatigue and severe difficulty concentrating on his teaching duties. For the four weeks before coming to the clinic, he found it increasingly difficult to wake up and he was late to class each morning. He felt that his energy level and mood were low. He said that he had this problem for as long as he could remember, but that it was a particular problem now because he had a new job and new responsibilities. He was having a hard time paying his bills, and his dishes had piled up in his sink. He was prescribed light therapy, which is exposure to a lamp that produces light of a certain intensity, thereby effectively extending daylight hours for the hapless teacher. This lifted his mood and he was able to continue through the winter without further problems.

It seems that the ancients recognized many of these symptoms. The biggest leap in our understanding comes from a much clearer sense of the brain and the chemicals that make the brain function.

BRAIN ANATOMY AND CHEMISTRY AS IT PERTAINS TO DEPRESSION

It is impossible to understand depression or how medication treatment works without having a basic sense of brain anatomy and the brain chemicals or neurotransmitters that allow the brain to function. One of the most consistent research findings is that a disturbance in neurotransmission or a so-called "chemical imbalance" is a hallmark of depression. Changes in the brains of depressed patients have been found in the following neurotransmitter systems: serotonin, norepinephrine, dopamine, corticotropin releasing factor (CRF), and somatostatin. The areas of the brain that are most relevant to depression are the frontal lobe and brainstem. Figure 2.1 provides a simple and basic look at the brain.

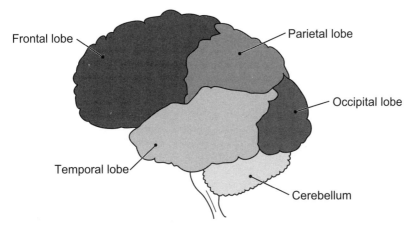

Figure 2.1. The human brain. *Illustrated by Jeff Dixon.*

If we now slice the brain in half, as we might an orange, we would see what appears in Figure 2.2. The brainstem is the lower part of the brain, or the part that connects the brain to the spinal cord. Inside the brainstem is a collection of nerves known as the raphe nuclei, which produce and release the neurotransmitter serotonin to the rest of the brain.

A part of the brain known as the locus ceruleus, which is under the cerebellum, produces most of the norepinephrine in the brain.

There is a group of nerve cells known as the substantia nigra, which lie deep within the brain and are responsible for most of the dopamine production.

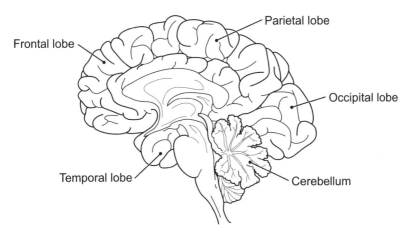

Figure 2.2. Schematic of a lengthwise cross-section through the human brain. *Illustrated by Jeff Dixon.*

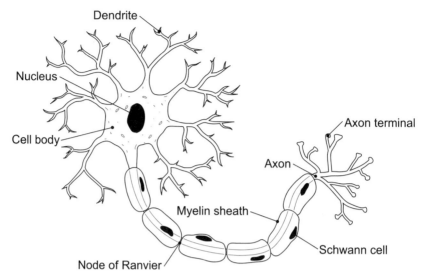

Figure 2.3. A typical brain nerve cell or neuron. *Illustrated by Jeff Dixon.*

Imbalances in neurotransmitters such as serotonin, dopamine, and norepinephrine have been linked to depression, and it is these imbalances that medications try to correct.

Another brain region linked to depression is the hypothalamus, which lies just above the brainstem. It regulates body temperature, blood pressure, heartbeat, metabolism of fats and carbohydrates, and sugar levels in the blood. CRF is an important hormone released by the hypothalamus and is considered important in the genesis of depression.

The brain is made up of specialized brain cells called neurons. It has been estimated that the brain contains 100 billion nerve cells or neurons. Figure 2.3 describes the structure and components of a typical neuron.

A message would travel from the dendrite through the cell body down the axon to the axon terminal and then into the synapse.

Dendrite→→→→→→→→→→Axon Terminal

Dendrites are the part of the neuron that collect information from other nerve cells and pass that information to the cell body. They look like the root network of a tree. A very important part of the whole neuron network is the space between the cell body of one neuron and the dendrite of another. This space is known as the synapse. The synapse plays a critical role in all brain function, and it is in this space that brain chemicals do their stuff, and it is in this space we need adequate levels of neurotransmitters for depression not to occur.

The cell body of the nerve cell is also known as the soma. It contains the cell nucleus, which produces all the proteins necessary for the functioning of the dendrites, axons, and synapses.

Axons are the main transmission lines of the brain. The axon is also known as the "nerve fiber." It carries messages away from the cell body toward the axon terminals. Neurons never physically touch. They communicate with each other across a tiny gap known as the synapse. The message is carried from the axon terminal of one cell to the dendrites of the next cell.

Neurotransmitters are the "brain chemicals." In nerve cells these chemicals are stored in tiny biological containers known as synaptic vesicles. They are released from these containers, which are located in the axon terminal of one cell, into the synapse or space between the cells. The neurotransmitter then keys into a receptor on the dendrite of the next cell. Neurotransmitters are like keys that fit into the receptor lock. The receptor will recognize only one type of neurotransmitter chemical, so that serotonin can only latch onto a se-rotonin receptor, dopamine to a dopamine receptor, and so on. It is these brain chemicals that are affected by antidepressant medication.

The Neurotransmitters of Depression

Serotonin plays an important role in the regulation of body temperature, mood, sleep, sexuality, and appetite. Low levels of serotonin have been shown in many studies to be associated with clinical depression and other conditions. Studies in which serotonin was depleted in the brain by reducing serotonin production precipitated symptoms of depression in healthy volunteers and in previously depressed patients who no longer suffered from depression. Also, postmortem studies have confirmed decreased serotonin in the brains of depressed patients and those who committed suicide.

Norepincphrinc (also known as noradrenaline) is a neurotransmitter that has many functions in the brain, including regulating attention and mood. Low epinephrine levels are thought to play a particularly important role in regulating the decreased drive and energy found in depression.

Epinephrine (also known as adrenaline) is a neurotransmitter closely related to norepinephrine. It is the "fight-or-flight" hormone and is released from the adrenal glands (which sit on top of the kidneys) when danger threat-ens. When released into the bloodstream, it quickly readies the body for action in emergency situations. The hormone boosts the supply of oxygen and energy-giving glucose to the brain and muscles. Some people have poorly regu-lated epinephrine regulation, and this can lead to severe anxiety and stress, both of which can lead to depression.

Dopamine is typically associated with the pleasure system of the brain and leads to the sense of enjoyment associated with certain activities such as eating, sex, and certain drug use. It plays a crucial role in processing motivation and reward. Dopamine is also involved in depression, and low levels of dopamine lead to marked lethargy. It has been shown that amphetamines (which increase dopamine in the brain) and dopamine reuptake blockers (which block the reuptake of dopamine thereby increasing the dopamine level) have potent antidepressant effects. However, these drugs quickly lose their effect as they lead to depletion of dopamine, which in turn leads to depression.

CRF is released from neurons in the hypothalamus, especially under conditions of stress. CRF sends a message to the adrenal glands, which in turn release cortisol. Under various stressful conditions, including exercise, trauma, anxiety, and depression, cortisol levels rise, leading to a chain of events that provides immediate energy to the body and keeps the individual alert. However, under prolonged stress, cortisol is constantly released, and this leads to serious physical consequences, including increased blood pressure, diabetes, arteriosclerosis, immune suppression, osteoporosis or bone breakdown, and muscle loss.

Understanding the symptoms of depression, as well as the workings of the brain and its chemistry, allows for a systematic approach to the diagnostic evaluation.

THE DIAGNOSTIC EVALUATION

The evaluation of a person suffering from depression consists of various steps. The usual procedure in psychiatry, as in all of medicine, is first to gather as much information as possible, then to establish a diagnosis, and finally to develop a treatment plan. In emergencies, this process is often modified because important data may not be available and the diagnosis is unclear. In emergencies, clinicians have to act immediately because waiting can have serious if not lethal consequences. The diagnostic process is best illustrated by considering a hypothetical case, and, for the purpose of completeness, I propose the case of a depressed, suicidal man.

Step 1: Obtaining the Clinical History, Including as Much of the Demographic Information as Possible

A white man who appeared to be in his 40s was brought by ambulance to the emergency room of a busy Boston hospital after his wife, Mary, found him at home slumped at his computer desk. She found a suicide note on the computer screen. By the time of his arrival at the emergency room, he was lethargic but awake and initially stated that he had taken sixty over-the-counter "sleeping pills." His wife stated that he was also on blood-pressure pills to control his hypertension and that she found the bottle empty by the computer. She also found a single empty beer bottle in the room.

Although drowsy, he was able to confirm his name (Michael), age (43), and address in south Boston. He admitted to planning his suicide attempt over the previous month. He lost his high-paying union job and felt that he was "a waste of human flesh, and a terrible husband and father."

His suicide note read, "Mary, I have failed you, my family and myself. I cannot see any way out of it. Maybe with the insurance money I will finally have given you what you all deserved. I'm sorry I could not find another way. Please give whatever organs I have that are still working for transplantation to someone who needs them."

Given the seriousness of his attempt and the clear intention in his note, the doctors ordered for a psychiatric worker to sit with Michael at all times throughout his stay in the emergency room so that he could be closely monitored.

Michael admitted to the emergency room doctors that he made a suicide attempt soon after he graduated from college, fell into a deep depression, and had been unable to hold a job. He acknowledged that he had been depressed for years and had seen a psychiatrist and a therapist on and off over the years but had not kept any appointments over the past eight months. He admitted that he had ongoing suicidal thoughts and seemed disappointed that he had not succeeded in dying, stating, "I'm pathetic, I can't do anything, I can't even kill myself."

Step 2: The Physical Examination

Although many psychiatrists do not personally perform a physical examination of their depressed patients, the physical exam is an essential part of the evaluation of the depressed patient. This is because, as we will see in the next chapter, there are many medical illnesses that can cause depression.

Michael's blood pressure was stable in the emergency room. His blood tests revealed that he was dehydrated. A drug screen revealed the presence of alcohol and a high, but not toxic, level of acetaminophen. Acetaminophen is a painkiller (the main ingredient in Tylenol) and is found in some over-the-counter sleep aids.

Although he was lethargic, his heart and lung examination was normal. He underwent nasogastric lavage, which is a procedure in which a plastic tube is placed through a patient's nose into their stomach to drain the contents of the stomach. The hope is to remove much of the medication that remains in the stomach before it can be absorbed by the small intestine. He was then treated with activated charcoal, which is a substance made essentially from charcoal. It has become the treatment of choice for many poisonings and works by attaching to the toxin to prevent stomach and intestinal absorption. Michael was admitted to the medical intensive care unit to monitor him for twenty-four hours to ensure that he remained clinically stable.

Step 3: The Psychiatric Evaluation

Given that there did not appear to be any significant medical complications to his overdose nor any other medical reasons for his depression, the psychiatry consultation liaison team was asked to see him. Michael continued to express suicidal thoughts, and the next day he was transferred to a locked inpatient psychiatric unit. Patients are placed on a locked unit when staff worry that they are a risk to themselves or others and if they worry that the person might run from the unit and end up hurting themselves or another person.

On the unit, the psychiatrist continued the evaluation of Michael, who admitted to hopelessness, helplessness, insomnia, decreased appetite with weight loss, and poor sleep. He complained of low self-esteem over the past six years, after initially being laid off from his job as a software engineer and then being unable to find steady work. He considered himself a failure as a father and a husband. He denied that he had ever heard voices in his head or that he had ever been abused. He denied ever having felt happy for extended periods of time. He denied ever having been hospitalized for a psychiatric problem but said that he had been treated on and off for depression in the past and that depression ran in his family. He said that a maternal uncle killed himself and that a first cousin on his mother's side also suffered from depression. He denied abusing any drugs and admitted that he enjoyed the occasional beer. On interviewing his wife, she endorsed all of his reports but further added that she was very worried because he appeared to have given up on himself and that he stopped caring for himself. He was bathing less frequently and often wore the same clothes for many days despite her pleas that he bathe and change.

Step 4: The Mental State Examination

Because there are presently no brain-imaging devices or machines that categorically diagnose psychiatric illness, the history and mental status examination (MSE) are the most important diagnostic tools a psychiatrist has to obtain the data necessary to make an accurate diagnosis.

The MSE is an assessment of a patient's level of cognitive ability, appearance, emotional mood, and speech and thought patterns at the time of evaluation. It includes the examiner's observations about the patient's attitude and cooperativeness as well as the patient's answers to specific questions. The specific components of the MSE for the patient are as follows:

1. Appearance: This is a record of the patient's physical appearance, sex, age, race, and ethnic background. In this hypothetical case, the psychiatrist would describe Michael as a disheveled (perhaps malodorous secondary to not showering) white male in his mid-40s.

2. Attitude toward the examiner: This is a record of the patient's facial expressions and attitude toward the examiner (such as whether the patient is bored, hostile, cooperative, or friendly). This part of the examination is based solely on observations made by the mental healthcare professional. Michael would be described as being reasonably cooperative.

3. Mood: This is a record of the patient's own description of their current mood. Michael described his mood as "depressed."

4. Affect: This is a record of the observations made by the interviewer during the course of the interview of a patient's affect and is defined in the following terms: expansive (contagious), euthymic (normal), constricted (limited variation), labile (rapidly changing), blunted (minimal variation), and flat (no variation). Michael's affect would be described as labile or constricted.

5. Speech: This is a record on all aspects of the patient's speech, including quality, quantity, rate, and volume of speech during the interview. Typical of depressed patients, Michael would probably have soft speech, with less spontaneity of speech than in a nondepressed patient.

6. Thought process: This is a record of the patient's thought process and is described in the following terms: looseness of association (irrelevance), flight of ideas (change topics), racing (rapid thoughts), tangential (departure from topic with no return), circumstantial (being vague), word salad (nonsensical responses), derailment (extreme irrelevance), neologism (creating new words), clanging (rhyming words), punning (talking in riddles), thought blocking (speech is halted), and poverty (limited content). The thought process of the depressed patient is often normal, unless they are psychotic; then they might make up words, change topics frequently, or have irrelevant answers to questions.

7. Thought content: This is a determination of whether or not a patient is experiencing hallucinations or delusions and whether there are obsessions and compulsions or phobias. Most important is to assess whether a person has suicidal or homicidal thoughts. Michael is

clearly having ongoing suicidal thoughts. He feels that he is a total failure and feels no hope that his life will change.

8. Sensorium and cognition: This is an assessment of a person's cognitive ability and examines their level of consciousness, degree of orientation to their current surroundings (does a patient know who he is, where they are, or what day it is?), concentration and attention, memory, abstract thinking, general fund of knowledge, and intelligence. Depressed patients tend to complain of a decrease in ability to attend and concentrate, and, in Michael's case, given the amount of medication he had taken, the psychiatrist would probably note that he was not fully alert.

9. Insight: This is an assessment of the patient's understanding of the illness. Michael appears to have good insight into the fact that he is depressed

10. Judgment: This is an assessment of the person's capacity for judgment. Sometimes this is done based on their response to an imaginary scenario such as "What would you do if you smelled smoke in a crowded theater?" Often the psychiatrist can assess a person's judgment based on their choice in a particular real-life event. Michael appears to show poor judgment (probably on the basis of his depression) in that he believes that the only way out for him is to kill himself.

Step 5: Other Tests

Although psychological testing is not essential in making a psychiatric diagnosis, at times when the picture is confusing, the psychiatrist may request such testing to corroborate the diagnosis.

Tests such as IQ testing to assess the person's intelligence on a standardized test or the Minnesota Multiphasic Personality Inventory-2 (MMPI-2) are often used. The MMPI was developed in the late 1930s by psychologist Starke R. Hathaway and psychiatrist J.C. McKinley at the University of Minnesota and is used to diagnose psychiatric illness. Despite being developed so long ago, it continues to be the most frequently used clinical testing instrument. The MMPI-2 is a newer version of the original. Another scale used specifically in depression is the Beck Depression Inventory (BDI). It is a self-administered twenty-one-item self-report scale measuring manifestations of depression. The BDI takes approximately ten minutes to complete, although clients require a fifth to sixth grade reading age to adequately understand the questions.

The scoring for the BDI is as follows for total score levels of depression: 0–4, either no problem or the person is faking; 5–9, these ups and downs are considered normal; 10–18, mild to moderate depression; 19–29, moderate to severe depression; 30–63, severe depression; over 40, either severe depression or an exaggeration of depression. Michael's BDI score was 32, indicating a severe depression.

At times, and even if the physical exam is normal, a physician may order a brain imaging scan such as a computerized tomography (CAT) scan or a magnetic resonance imaging scan. In Michael's case, given that he was drowsy and had a history of high blood pressure, the clinicians could justifiably worry about his having had a small stroke. Michael's head CAT scan showed no abnormalities.

Diagnostic Formulation and Treatment Plan

Given the completeness of Michael's evaluation, he can be fairly reliably diagnosed as suffering from severe depression with ongoing suicidal thoughts but without clear evidence of psychotic thinking.

The treatment plan included Michael's initial admission to a locked psychiatric unit. This was done to keep him on a suicide watch because he remained depressed and had ongoing thoughts of suicide. Next a decision would be made as to medication and would take into account symptoms such as sleep (does he need a sedating antidepressant or not), previous trials of medications, previous side effects to medications, concern over whether he might have bipolar disorder (when the use of an antidepressant might make him manic), co-occurring medical conditions (some antidepressants case high blood pressure), and other medications the person might be taking. The decision to use medication, however, generally depends on the outcome of the evaluation. There are a variety of antidepressant medications and psychotherapies used to treat depressive disorders. Some people with milder forms may do well with psychotherapy alone. People with moderate to severe depression most often benefit from antidepressants. Most patients do best with a combination of medication to gain relatively quick symptom relief and psychotherapy to learn more effective coping in dealing with life's problems.

Given the severity of Michael's depression, he is a good candidate for both medication and therapy and would therefore be assigned to a therapist and group therapy sessions within the unit, while at the same time the team would work toward establishing an outpatient team that would continue to provide therapy and follow his progress after his discharge from the hospital. Three weeks after starting medication, Michael showed some signs of improvement. His appetite, sleep, and personal hygiene all improved. He began to talk about his future hopes and began to make calls for potential job interviews. He appeared more relaxed around his wife. Finally, he acknowledged that he no longer had suicidal thoughts, although he was worried that they might return. He had a few passes back to his home and to meet his outpatient team and was finally discharged from the hospital.

In the case of our hypothetical Michael, an evaluation and formulation led to good treatment and a good outcome. Michael, however, was a forty-something white male. In the next few sections, we will look at how gender, race, and age affect the picture of clinical depression.

The above was the evaluation of a hypothetical Michael, but the procedure would have been the same for a hypothetical female patient Michaela. Although men and women share identical brain chemistry and neuroanatomy, many have wondered whether the female brain is different from the male brain. It is certainly true that men and women experience and react to depression in different ways. The American comedian Elayne Boosler once quipped on Comedy Central, "When women are depressed, they eat or go shopping. Men invade another country. It's a whole different way of thinking."

DEPRESSION AND GENDER

Universally, depression is at least twice as common in women as in men. In the United States, depression is the main cause of disability in women. Women also have higher rates of seasonal affective disorder, depressive symptoms in bipolar disorder, and dysthymia. Women experience guilt, anxiety, increased appetite and sleep, and weight gain more frequently than men do. Statistics show that, in their lifetime, depression will affect 10–25 percent of women and 5–12 percent of men. At any one point in time, 5–9 percent of all women and 2–3 percent of all men are likely to be clinically depressed.

So why is it that women have more depression than men? A common argument goes that women receive a diagnosis of depression more often than men because men are less likely to acknowledge the symptoms and that, instead, depressed men become angry and irritable or drink heavily. Also, men are less likely to seek professional help. However, statistics show that women have higher rates of depression even in surveys of people who have never sought mental health treatment.

There have been many attempts to explain why women experience depression at higher rates than men. One explanation is women's exposure to stress. Women suffer from certain types of severe stress (abuse, violence) and less severe stress (balancing work and family) than men do, and women are three times more likely than men to become depressed in response to a stressful event. Stress and, in particular, severe stress leads to brain chemistry changes that lead to depression.

The issue of the consideration of gender in depression preceded the age of statistics. Hildegard von Bingen was born in 1098 in Nahe, Germany, and was the tenth child of Hildebert and Mechthild von Bermersheim who were minor nobility of the Holy Roman Empire. At eight years of age, she was entrusted to Jutta, an anchoress or hermit who spent her life in prayer and solitude. From Jutta, Hildegard would learn Latin and religion. Hildegard devoted herself to the religious life and became a nun. After Jutta's death, Hildegard would go on to run a small convent, and she became a prolific author, musician, counselor, artist, healer, linguist, naturalist, philosopher, poet, religious consultant, and visionary.

In the 1150s, Hildegard completed the book *Causae et Curae* or *Of Causes and Cures*. It reflected a "knowledge of the popular and monastic practices of its day, as well as Hildegard's own personal experience not only as a sufferer but also as one who herself attended and healed the sick" (Radden 2000).

In her book, she described "the Melancholic" as a person who is dour, nervous, and changeable in their mood. She too concurred with the idea that melancholy was caused by black bile, which she believed was caused by the first attack of the devil on Adam, and that this would curse Adam and all of his descendants. She wrote that melancholy affected men and women differently. Of men, she wrote that their brains were fat and that their scalp and blood vessels were entangled. She described their eyes as having something serpentine-like about them. They had large bones but little marrow. Their behavior with women was improper and as undisciplined as wild animals. They love no one and are embittered, resentful, and are as "unregulated in their interactions with women as a donkey" (Radden 2000). If they abstained from sex, they could easily become sick in the head. "Some of them traffic enthusiastically, in the male way, with women because they have strong blood vessels and marrow that burns mightily in them, however afterwards they hate these women. In practical matters however, they are skillful and enjoy working."

Of women, she wrote that melancholic women had "thin flesh, thick blood vessels, and moderately strong bones." She wrote that they were "heedless of evil disposition and grieved by any irritation." During menses, these women would lose much blood and be infertile because of a weak womb, and this prevented them from receiving the "male seed." She argued that these women were happier without a mate than with one and that they would become sick from having sex with their husband. Hildegard said that these women were avoided in any case because they did not speak in a friendly manner to men and that any desire of the flesh appeared to go away quickly. Another symptom was that, if the melancholic woman stopped having her menses, she would become arthritic and have kidney problems and swollen legs and that, without God's help, would die.

Hildegard regarded men's presentation of depression to be marked by uncontrollable and undisciplined sexual desires. Women's depression, on the other hand, was characterized by irritability, antisocial behavior, and physical symptoms. Clearly Hildegard had given the distinction on the matter much thought. Whether or not men's undisciplined sexual desires or women's inability to receive the male seed have anything to do with depression is pertinent in that, in women, an important treatment consideration is pregnancy, or the consideration of pregnancy as the potential effects of antidepressants on a fetus or newborn might need to be considered.

Another factor important in female depression is hormonal. Premenstrual dysphoric disorder is a severe form of premenstrual syndrome occurring in 2–10 percent of menstruating women. It appears to be caused by the hormonal changes that take place around menses and is characterized by depressed mood, anxiety, tension, and irritability. Sadly, the mood changes of the premenstrual period have all too often not been given sufficient medical recognition and at times become subject of jokes, as pointed out in Adrienne Wardy's paper *I Have PMS and a Handgun, Any Questions?: Demystifying the Definition, Causes, and Treatment of PMS and PMDD*.

Pregnancy and the postpartum phase also contribute to the increased incidence of depression in women. Studies show that about 10–20 percent of pregnant women suffer from antepartum depression (depression during pregnancy) and that 10–15 percent of mothers become depressed during the first six months after childbirth. Poverty, single motherhood, an unwanted pregnancy, and a temperamentally difficult baby exacerbate depression. Despite this, wealth or fame does not protect from postpartum depression.

Brooke Shields for one says, "The very damaging, frightening part of postpartum is the lack of perspective and the lack of priority and understanding what is really important." Marie Osmond once warned, "This is a serious, serious condition that is also called postpartum psychosis. And that's where, literally, you get so bad that you end up either hurting the baby or killing yourself." In Europe, this risk is considered so real that, if it occurs, it is often not criminalized. In English law (the Infanticide Act of 1938), a mother who kills her child within the first year of the child's life is assumed to be mentally ill. The highest crime she can be charged with is manslaughter, and English juries are reluctant to sentence women to prison for this crime, although fathers can be charged with homicide.

American law classifies infanticide as a homicide. Depending on state laws, those who commit infanticide may be eligible for the death penalty. The most notorious of such cases in America was that of Marie Noe who, between 1949 and 1968, had ten children, seven girls and three boys. None of her children lived to see their second birthday. She claimed that they had all died while sleeping of sudden infant death syndrome. Although the Philadelphia investigators were suspicious, they found no evidence of foul play but, at age 70, she finally admitted that she had smothered eight of the babies and pleaded guilty to eight counts of second-degree murder.

For women unable to get pregnant, infertility problems are a great risk for stress, severe anxiety, and sadness, and those going through infertility treatments are subject to large hormonal changes, which can lead to irritability and depression.

Stress and anxiety contribute to and aggravate depression. Women often bear the responsibility of juggling the demands of home and work, at times having to coordinate care for their children, aging parents, and home life. Women are also more likely to face the responsibility of caring for their children as single parents. Major depression is highest among the separated and divorced for both men and women, yet even in this group it is still higher overall for women. The quality of a marriage contributes significantly to depression, so lack of intimacy and trust and constant marital disputes are related to depression in women. Rates of depression in unhappily married women are much higher than those in unhappily married men.

Whatever the type of depression and whether it is man or woman, depression is a serious condition that takes its toll on the quality and, at times, the actuality of life. William Styron, the author of *Darkness Visible*, describes this best when he says, "In depression ... faith in deliverance, in ultimate restoration, is absent. The pain is unrelenting, and what makes the condition intolerable is the foreknowledge that no remedy will come—not in a day, an hour, a month, or a minute.... It is hopelessness even more than pain that crushes the soul."

Given the differences between how men and women experience depression, perhaps it should not be surprising that marked cultural differences exist as well.

CULTURE, RELIGION, AND DEPRESSION

Karima was an attractive eighteen-year-old woman who had been brought to the emergency room by her aunt and uncle for "not feeling well." She said through a translator that she had been born in Germany of first-generation Moroccan parents. She had arrived in the United States only two months earlier hoping to make a life for herself and was living with her aunt and uncle, who were Muslim. Her parents were hoping to make their way to

America as soon as they raised enough money. She also left behind a younger sister, and a third sister had died of unspecified "brain problems." After her physical exam and blood tests failed to reveal any clear problem, she was referred to our psychiatric service for a consultation. Once again, with the aid of a skilled translator, Karima said that she was troubled by feelings of sadness, insomnia, guilt, loneliness, and worthlessness and that she had started having thoughts of death. These DSM-IV symptoms of major depression had appeared nearly three weeks earlier according to her family and were consistent with Karima hearing that her parents were not going to come to America anytime soon. Karima had never suffered psychiatric problems before, and the family was skeptical of a diagnosis of depression.

Her aunt and uncle had some cultural explanations for what was physically happening to Karima. They stated that, about a year before her arrival in the United States, she had been invited to a wedding in Morocco. According to them, the bride's parents had seen Karima as an exotic rival to the bride. They further suggested that someone could have thrown the evil eye on Karima to protect the bride. Another cultural explanation was sorcery. Her aunt wondered whether the spirit of Karima's younger sister, who had died of the "brain problem," could be in Karima's body. Karima herself struggled between the "depression" explanation that the psychiatrist was giving her through the translator and her family's views on the problem. The family left the emergency room with a plan to meet with a psychiatrist in the outpatient clinic the next day. It took two more weeks of Karima's symptoms for the family finally to agree to a trial of antidepressant medication and therapy. It took an additional five weeks for her symptoms to lift.

The DSM-IV criteria for major depression were reviewed earlier in this chapter. Although the DSM criteria for depression may resonate as being a true and accurate picture of the condition, millions of people would neither recognize the condition as depression nor treat it the same way. In fact, major depression has a wide cultural variation.

Webster's Third New International Unabridged Dictionary defines culture as "the total pattern of human behavior and its products embodied in thought, speech, action, and artifacts and dependent upon man's capacity for learning and transmitting knowledge to succeeding generations through the use of tools, language, and systems of abstract thought." Today, mental health professionals are often called on to provide culturally competent care in dealing with patients from a wide variety of cultures. Such challenges are especially significant for healthcare providers in gateway cities or points of arrival in the United States. These challenges are also true for "Western" trained mental health staff working with Native American populations.

Many impoverished immigrant Asian, African, and Latino people suffering under the burden of poverty, unemployment, alienation, and loneliness and who develop depression present in emergency rooms with various complaints generally physical in nature. If a consideration of a mental problem is offered, many foreign immigrants refuse to consider the possibility, often attributing the problem to "evil spirits." This attribution of the problem to spirits is often true irrespective of culture, although the actual name for the problem may be different in each culture.

Hispanic Americans sometimes label their depression as an "ataque de nervios," literally an "attack of the nerves." Symptoms of an ataque can include crying, trembling, excessive worry, dissociative experiences, fainting episodes, and suicidal gestures.

Very religious Hispanic and Asian communities will often confuse hallucinations with spiritual voices and look to their priest and ministers for religious cures. In the cases in which these interventions are not enough, there is often great shame in both seeking out mental health help or being seen at a mental health clinic.

The understanding of depression can vary between cultures and religions or depend on educational status. The following descriptions are a sample of the remarkable diversity in the conceptualization of depression.

Buddhism and Depression

> On occasion, without any special external event taking place, there can simply be a dysfunction or disruption in the balance of the elements within the body. In that event, the internal circumstances are the dominant, principal cause.
>
> (the Dalai Lama)

The Buddhist view of how the mind works is different from the traditional Western view. Western psychology has generally held the belief that emotions are hard to change. Buddhism believes that emotions can be readily controlled through the practice of specific skills. This view is strongly supported by neuroscience, which has provided evidence of the brain's capacity for change and growth.

Buddhism uses meditation to control the emotions. Interestingly, some Western psychologists are increasingly adopting this perspective and seeing depression as a disorder of emotional mismanagement. In this view, a person's awareness is overwhelmed by negative events and then sets off a kind of chain reaction of negative feeling, thinking, and behavior. Reclaiming awareness permits the cultivation of self-control and allows a person to break the negative emotional chain reaction and head off the hopelessness and despair that results.

One meditative practice is to use breathing techniques in which the focus is on the breathing and which lets any negative thoughts simply "go by" rather than bringing them into the mind and allowing them to play over and over, magnifying the negativity of such thoughts. It is therefore a way of unlearning the self-defeating behavior learned previously as a response to negative experiences.

Medications are sometimes used to jump-start the brain but are described as "a halfway house" by psychologist Alan Wallace, Ph.D., head of the Santa Barbara Institute for the Study of Consciousness. The Buddhist idea that changing depression and controlling the mind by reclaiming awareness is best summed up in a quote from the Buddha himself: "We are shaped by our thoughts; we become what we think. When the mind is pure, joy follows like a shadow that never leaves."

Islam and Depression

Clinical descriptions of depression by Muslim psychiatrists are essentially identical to such descriptions by Western psychiatrists.

Many orthodox and religious Muslims, however, do not recognize the concept of depression and feel that a "true" Muslim cannot suffer from this "disease." The Koran emphatically says: "Every soul shall have a taste of death: and We test you by evil and by good by way of trial. To Us must you return" (Koran 21:35). It also points out: "No burden do We place on any soul, but that which it can bear" (Koran 6:152).

Writer Muhammad Zafar Adeel states, "The answer lies in this fundamental understanding, which governs a Muslim's life: his life with all its ups and downs is a trial." He argues that, for a true Muslim, difficulties in life are as vital for the continuation of life as is oxygen for breathing, that each incident has both a bright side and a dull side to it. It is part of a Muslim's faith that Allah knows everything that lies ahead and that a strong faith in the Almighty promises a more desirable and everlasting reward in the Hereafter. Despite the perspective that difficulties are a part of life, Adeel recognizes that it is also important to understand that seeking help in times of despair is something that God would expect from His believers. He points out that even the great Prophets called on God's help in times of gloom. For instance, the Prophet Jacob says, "I only complain of my distraction and anguish to God" (Koran 12:86).

Because of the "nonexistence" of the concept of depression as a clinical condition and rather the idea that it is simply a trial of life, "treatment" of the devout Muslim who experiences depression involves prayer and the deepening of their faith in God.

An African Perspective

The Baganda people of Uganda conceptualize the symptoms associated with depression as a problems related to cognition or "thinking too much" rather than thinking of it as a problem of emotions such as sadness. They consider depression to be an "illness of thoughts," requiring no medication because it is believed that there is no medication for thoughts. The illness is generated because the sufferer has somehow upset the spirit world.

The spirit world of the Baganda dominates their perspective on health. The occupants of the spirit world inhabit three levels. The first is Katonda (the supreme creator), then the Lubaale, and then the Mizimu or the ancestral ghosts. The Lubaale or the godly spirits, of whom there are more than two dozen, are of major significance. They are guardians of the living but could cause illness when offended. However, of more day-to-day importance to the ordinary folk are the innumerable lesser spirits, the Mizimu. They are thought to be mostly benevolent, but some are known to be maliciously harmful if not kept happy. Rituals aimed at ensuring the goodwill of all spirits are part of everyday Baganda life.

When the "illness of thoughts" occurs, the Baganda believe that, because the problem is one of disharmony with the spirit world, treatment occurs through intercession with the spirit world. Traditional healers, who prescribe traditional rituals, are a preferred source of help for the "illness of thought" problem. In fact, taking the patient to the hospital is considered a waste of time.

For the Baganda, if the depression also has psychotic thinking such as delusions or hallucinations, the condition is known as eByekika or "Clan illness," and is considered to be caused by actions or behavior of the living toward the dead, such as the neglect of traditional rituals, breaking taboos, or mixing African and Western belief systems.

A Japanese Perspective

Tadashi Onda, a Japanese psychiatrist, said in a *New York Times* interview, "In a culture of shame, the only thing to do about illnesses of the mind is to hide them. They still carry a stigma here that can haunt families down through the generations. The best parallel I can imagine is the war, when tens of thousands of Japanese soldiers preferred dying in hopeless circumstances rather than surrendering—because of the power of shame" (French 2002).

Researchers in Japan have compared notes with their American counterparts on the symptoms of depression in Japanese and American depressed patients. They found that people with depression in Japan presented with more physical symptoms than those in the United States. Because of the "physical presentation" of the depression in Japanese patients, primary care

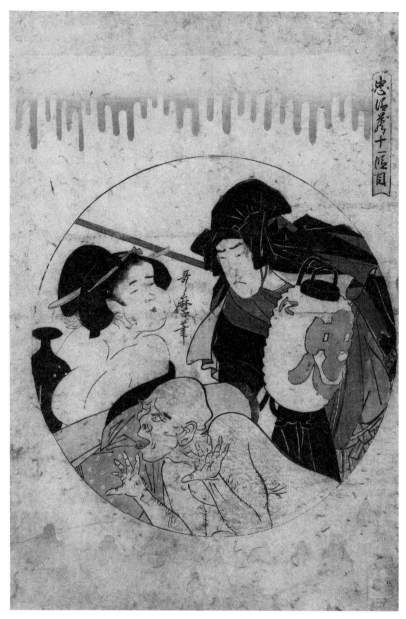

Figure 2.4. Print of a depressed old man, a warrior carrying a lantern, and the Japanese goddess of joy, Otafuku. *Courtesy Library of Congress, Prints & Photographs Division, LC-DIG-jpd-00194.*

doctors rarely diagnose depression in Japan but rather look for the causes of this physical illness. Even when no organic cause for the "physical symptoms" can be found, depression is often still not diagnosed.

In his interview, Onda continues, "Thirty thousand people commit suicide in Japan every year, but if we could diagnose them and treat them, in time that number would go down dramatically. I've never even heard of anyone specializing in depression, though. The bigger problem in Japan is that a stigma attaches to anyone seen as treating crazy people, and the status of psychiatrists remains very low."

Japanese culture is considered to play an important part in the choice of three areas of the body for the physical expression of depression, and people generally choose a doctor according to the organ they think is bothering them. The main symptoms with which depressed Japanese patients presented were abdominal (stomach) symptoms, neck/shoulder pain, and headaches.

Many Japanese expressions use the word "hara," or abdomen, to verbalize emotion. These include "hara ga tatu" (provoking), "hara guroi" (wicked), or "hara gei" (depending on the heart for understanding). In Japanese, "hara" (abdomen) is considered to be the place where ideas and feelings are located.

"Kanpo" is a traditional form of Japanese medicine. A "kanpo" doctor often uses the traditional procedure "Sesshin" (touching diagnosis) to diagnose the nature of an imbalance in the patient's body. Touching the abdomen is the most important examination. Because of the cultural association of the abdomen with emotions and the high number of medical visits for digestive system problems, it is understandable that depressed Japanese patients would present their psychological distress as an abdominal problem.

Neck and shoulder pain, or "katakori," is also a common reason for outpatient visits. Katakori is very loosely translated as a "pain in the neck" and, like the aforementioned abdominal pain, it is an expression of psychological distress with no obvious physical cause.

Interestingly, the Japanese often associate the word for depression, "yu-utsu," with external phenomena, such as rain or clouds, or with somatic symptoms, such as headaches. However, Japanese Americans generally associate the same word with terms such as sadness and loneliness. This change in how "yu-utsu" is conceptualized indicates that culture influences the presentation of depression. Over recent years, Western views of depression have been incorporated into Japanese culture so that young patients are far more likely to seek treatment today than their parents were in their generation.

A Chinese Perspective

A fifty-six-year-old Chinese woman, a recent immigrant to the United States, presented to a Seattle emergency room complaining of a "painful heart."

Immediately she had a comprehensive cardiac workup with an electrocardio-gram, full examination, and blood work. In Chinese, there is no word for depres-sion per se. The Chinese concept is translated as a "heavy heart" or a "painful heart." A purely "emotional" consideration of depression is generally dismissed.

Despite the dismissal of a Western view of depression, one statistic cannot be dismissed. Officially, around 250,000 people kill themselves in China every year. For young people between fifteen and thirty-four years of age, suicide is the main cause of death. Overall, it is the fifth most common cause of death in China after lung cancer, traffic accidents, heart disease, and other illnesses. Clearly, emotional problems are an issue, and, for these, many Chinese turn to Traditional Chinese Medicine (TCM).

In TCM, emotions and physical health are intimately connected. The Western psychological concepts of sadness, anxiety, anger, worry, and fear are each associated with a particular organ in the body. Depression is commonly referred to as "Yu Zheng" and is thought to affect the so-called Zang organs, which are the heart, lungs, liver, kidneys, and spleen. The heart is believed to store the spirit, which includes emotional reactions to stimuli. TCM further holds that each of the organs plays a role in emotions. The spleen is associated with excessive worry, the liver with anger, the kidneys with fear, and the lungs with anxiety and grief. As with ancient concepts of depression, which consid-ered imbalances in the body humors, so TCM believes that, when there is a disturbance in one or more of the Zang organs, an imbalanced emotional state including depression can occur. The Zang organs most frequently affected are the liver and the lungs.

Another fundamental concept in TCM is that of Qi. Qi or Chi is believed to be part of every living thing. It is loosely translated as a "life force" or "spir-itual energy." TCM believes that, when Qi is deficient and phlegm accumu-lates, energy cannot flow throughout the body. TCM therefore categorizes depression according to the organ affected.

Lung depression presents as an inability to let go of worries, shortness of breath, fatigue, sweating easily upon exertion, exhaustion, and soft or no speech. Physical findings include a pale tongue and a weak pulse. Liver depres-sion presents irritable and changing mood, poor appetite, abdominal pain, muscular tension, fatigue, and bowel problems. Physical findings also show a pale tongue and weak pulse. Then, if Qi and phlegm are not in harmony, depression presents with a gagging sensation and tightness in the chest. If the Zang organs are deficient in blood, this can present in a depression with feel-ings of restlessness, weepiness, fatigue, and chest tightness. Excessive phlegm presents as a depression with an inability to think clearly and concentrate, lack of appetite, and difficulty waking up in the morning.

Once the TCM practitioner has diagnosed the type of depression, TCM procedures such as acupuncture or medicines consisting of herbs and herb combinations are chosen to target the patient's symptoms.

Depression in African-American Women

African-American women often experience depression as ongoing and relentless symptoms. The presentation of depression is usually that of persistent, untreated physical and emotional symptoms. Depression is often the last symptom addressed by clinicians for these women who are frequently diagnosed as being hypertensive, run down, or tense and nervous. They may be prescribed blood pressure pills, vitamins, or painkillers, or they may be told to lose weight, learn to relax, or get more exercise. The root of their symptoms is generally not explored, and these women might continue to complain of being tired, weary, empty, lonely, and sad.

Unfortunately, a comprehensive psychiatric evaluation is much less common for depressed African-American women than for Caucasian American women. Furthermore, the offer of psychotherapy is just as uncommon. One reason given for the lower rate of diagnosis and therapy for African-American women is that they are the least likely group to commit suicide and so the diagnosis of depression or at least a severe depression is less likely, and an important treatment opportunity is missed.

Depression in Native Americans

Catherine Cheechoo of the Nishnawbe Aski Nation expressed the following in writing about the epidemic of suicide in the Native American population: "So much trauma and loss has been experienced within our communities, and we live with this every day. If you were to ask us why someone is contemplating suicide, you would get a variety of answers. The burden of issues we face in everyday life and the confusion while we attempt to sort it out is very tiring. Ultimately, it's the overwhelming sense of isolation, confusion, hopelessness, and sadness that leads to someone contemplating and attempting suicide. You may question how we know this—these feelings and the causes—and we would put it simply: we have experienced it. We may not know all the academic reasoning and ideology surrounding why people become suicidal, but what we do know is from our personal experiences in our communities and homes" (www.voicesforchildren.ca).

Researchers have attempted to measure the occurrence of major depression in Native Americans for many years. Unfortunately, there are still no good statistics. One statistic is, however, patently clear and that is that the suicide rate in the American Indian population is generally higher and is characterized by younger people engaging in fatal and nonfatal suicidal behavior at much higher rates than the overall U.S. population. Specifically, U.S. government data show that, for five to fourteen year olds, the suicide rate for American Indians is 2.6 times higher than the national average and, for fifteen to twenty-four year olds is 3.3 times higher than the national average. Despite these suicide facts, an adequate assessment of major depression in this population remains elusive. There is concern among researchers about just how useful Western measures of depression are when assessing American Indian populations due to vast differences in cultural beliefs about mental illness, cultural labeling of different emotions, and conceptual language differences. The symptoms of depression tend to be expressed as a cultural metaphor, such as a person complaining of having a "heavy heart" or "an esteem problem," or suffering a "lack of balance" or having problems considered simply to be a part of life.

Mental health professionals recognize that the American Indian populations are at great risk for depression, if they use risk factors for depression in Western populations. For instance, due to the remoteness and isolation of many communities, families experience disruptions such as enforced attendance at boarding schools, adoption, and fly-out hospitalizations for long-term illnesses. There is a major problem with alcohol and drug use within the communities, which perpetuate the misery. Studies of Native Americans who have committed suicide have found that as many as 90 percent of victims had alcohol in their blood. Brain damage or paranoid psychosis as a result of the chronic use of solvents is reported as a major factor in suicides by youths.

Socioeconomic factors, such as high rates of poverty, low levels of education, limited employment opportunities, inadequate housing, and deficiencies in sanitation and water quality, affect Native Americans disproportionately. These factors again compound the feelings of helplessness and hopelessness that can lead to suicide. Overlying all the above problems is the finding that a "cultural stress" permeates Native American life. This cultural stress is based on the historical loss of cultural identity, loss of land, loss of control over living conditions, suppression of belief systems and spirituality, weakening of social and political institutions, and racial discrimination.

Quite what depression is in Native American populations may be neither well understood nor clearly defined. The fact that suicide is so prevalent as a solution to the ever-present misery underscores the profound need for culturally competent mental health providers and a pressing need to address the many underlying sociopolitical and structural problems the communities face.

Depression in Latinos

Our psychiatry service was asked to see a thirty-two-year-old Puerto Rican mother of three young children who presented to the emergency room complaining of an "ataque de nervios." Her symptoms were depression, seeing spirits, poor appetite, memory problems, and feelings of sadness. She admitted that she had gone to see a spiritual healer for the same problem about a month earlier, although she also said that at that time her symptoms included stomach aches, sleep problems, and fear. Her spiritualist had laid hands on her, which took away the stomachaches, but the rest of her problems persisted and she wanted "help." She admitted also that she was under a lot of stress because one of her children was sick with asthma and that her husband had recently lost his job.

DSM-IV recognizes the existence of culture-bound syndromes. Relevant examples of these syndromes for Latinos are "susto" (fright), "ataque de nervios" (a nervous attack), and "mal de ojo" (evil eye). Not all Latinos experience these equally. For instance, Caribbean Latinos have more frequent "ataque de nervios" (Guarnaccia, De La Cancela, and Carrillo 1989). Symptoms of an "ataque de nervios" include screaming uncontrollably, crying, trembling, and verbal or physical aggression. Fainting episodes and suicidal gestures can be prominent in some "ataques de nervios."

However, not every Latino who complains of "nerves" should be considered as having a mental health problem. For instance, many people of Mexican origin apply the more general concept of "ataque de nervios" to general stress in their lives not associated with DSM disorders, as well as to distress that is associated with clinical anxiety and depression (Salgado de Snyder, Diaz-Perez, and Ojeda 2000). We see that depression is not only experienced differently between cultures but also that, even within a culture, a common language is not enough to guarantee a shared experience of the condition. Finally, as we will see, age too makes a difference.

DEPRESSION ACROSS THE LIFESPAN

Depression in Children and Teens: One End of the Spectrum

Adolescence

I'm seventeen and I'm crazy. My uncle says the two always go together. When people ask your age, he said, always say seventeen and insane.
                                        (Clarisse McClellan, quoted in Bradbury 1953)

Adolescence is a time of tremendous growth at many levels and often a time of great confusion for parents, especially as they face the normal developmental changes of their teens. Normal adolescents are frequently moody. Up until the teen years, children tend to see their parents as generally doing the right thing. They are certain at least that their parents know what they are doing, but, as adolescence approaches, the kids begin to recognize that their parents are not perfect, and they show less overt affection and at times rudeness toward them. Mark Twain once famously quipped, "When I was a boy of fourteen, my father was so ignorant I could hardly stand to have the old man around. But when I got to be twenty-one, I was astonished at how much the old man had learned in seven years" (Twain 1998, 27).

As kids begin to move toward independence, struggling with a sense of identity is common. They can tend to feel awkward or strange about their body, especially during the marked changes that come with the onset of puberty. They tend to focus on self, alternating between high expectations of their capabilities and poor self-esteem. They focus on clothing style, which is often influenced by their peer group as well as popular culture.

Very Young Children

However, even before reaching adolescence, depression may be present. Dr. James C. MacIntyre, an associate professor of psychiatry at Albany Medical College in New York, has pointed out that "First-graders can and do get depressed. It's not a common thing, but kids in the early grades experience significant depression" (www.webmd.com). He has cautioned that, on rare occasions, preschoolers can show signs of depression: "A child who stops playing with friends, or frequently complains of stomachaches or headaches or is considered a 'troublemaker' may actually be depressed."

One problem with studying depression in very young children is that a six-year-old T-ball player cannot possibly be evaluated in the same way as a seventeen-year-old sexually active, substance-using football player. The brain pathways of very young children are profoundly different from those of older teenagers, whose brains more closely resemble adult brains. Also, young children metabolize drugs differently from older teens or adults. This leads many psychiatrists to be very reluctant to prescribe drugs for younger children, although the practice does occur. Researchers continue to work on understanding how and why young children get depressed, and, as in adults, the early findings are pointing to a combination of genetic, biological, and environmental factors.

Normal Adolescence

In normal adolescence, there is frequent rule and limit testing at both home and school. It is also a time of increasing interest in sexuality, and most typically adolescents display shyness, easy embarrassment, and modesty, despite an increased interest in sex. There is generally a move toward heterosexuality and fears of homosexuality, and they are frequently preoccupied with concerns regarding their physical and sexual attractiveness to others. There also tends to be frequent changes in relationships. All these changes and behaviors are normal, but, other behaviors, such as in the story of James, can indicate the presence of a major depression.

I was recently asked to see James, a fifteen-year-old tenth grader, whom his parents described as having been an average student and good athlete who spent much of his free time playing video games or skateboarding with his friends. Things changed over the past eight months as he became increasingly moody, appeared depressed, and became more withdrawn to the point that he now rarely played video games or skateboarded with his friends. At first, his parents thought that this was just a part of normal adolescent development, but, as his mood deteriorated, they became increasingly worried. He had started dating a girl about four months earlier, but she left him as he became increasingly withdrawn, and this sent him into what his parents described as a "tailspin."

His sleep worsened and he started complaining of vague aches and would skip occasional school days. He refused to talk to his parents about what was going on. His father shared that his own father had suffered from depression and been hospitalized at one time for having suicidal thoughts. It was when they found a web page that James printed out on ways of committing suicide that they took him to his pediatrician, who in turn referred him for an evaluation.

In our meeting, James admitted that he had been feeling rageful that his girlfriend leaving him had made him want to kill himself, and feeling that he would never feel happy again. It was clear that James had slipped into a major depression and that he was at risk given his family history. Furthermore, his breakup with his girlfriend was a trigger for him, something we find in many adolescents who suffer from depression.

Depression in Teenagers

An alarming and increasing number of teenagers attempt and succeed at suicide. Suicide is the third leading cause of death in adolescents, and children as young as five have been reported to have committed suicide! Some researchers feel that suicide statistics for teens are underreported, because adolescents are often involved in reckless or dangerous behavior resulting in death, and many teens so behaving are suffering from clinical depression.

Unfortunately, depression in teens can look like normal adolescent moodiness because occasional bad moods and short periods of feeling down are common in adolescence. Major depression, however, limits an adolescent's ability to function normally. Depression in teenagers is characterized by a persistent sad mood, irritability, feelings of hopelessness, or the inability to feel pleasure or happiness for an extended period of time. Early symptoms of adolescent depression can be difficult to diagnose because they can appear to be a normal part of the developmental challenges of adolescence, and yet many teen behaviors or attitudes that are annoying to adults are actually indications of depression. The following symptoms are often considered as a sign that a depression may be brewing. The first includes changes in eating and sleeping habits that are not associated with a diet or need to "pull all-nighters" to get a paper completed. Another is missing school and or a sudden worsening in school performance and in grades, feeling a tremendous lack of motivation to get work completed, or feeling that nothing is worth the effort. Another classical symptom is withdrawal from friends and family, including no longer enjoying formerly fun hobbies and activities. This can sometimes be aggravated by the use of drugs and alcohol in an attempt to treat the feelings of hopelessness and isolation. Other than drug use, self-destructive behaviors such as self-injury and eating disorders such as anorexia and bulimia can be an indication of depression. Persistent feelings of worthlessness or guilt and an overreaction to criticism would be a worrisome sign. Teens with depression often have marked irritability, which can sometimes spill over into rage attacks and fights. Ultimately, as in all forms of depression, suicidal thinking and suicidal behavior are the most serious concerns complicating childhood and teen depression.

Teens and Suicide

In the past twenty-five years, although the general incidence of suicide has decreased, the rate for those between fifteen and twenty-four has tripled. It is generally considered to be the second or third most common cause of death among adolescents. Each year, about 20 percent of adolescents consider suicide, many seriously so; by the end of high school, one in ten has attempted it. About half of those who die suffer from major clinical depression. The fact of teen suicide is a tragedy; the fact that these deaths are underreported is yet another tragedy.

How Prevalent Is Childhood Depression?

It was only in the late 1980s that mental health clinicians gave any serious consideration to childhood depression. Before this, the condition was considered to be very rare, different from adult depression, and not treatable with antidepressants.

Today, approximately 5 percent of children and adolescents are experiencing a depression, with the percentage increasing with age. During childhood, the number of boys and girls is the same. However, in adolescence, girls outnumber boys 2-to-1, a ratio that continues into adulthood. Not all children and teens have the same risk of developing depression. Children with a family history of depression have a greater chance. So do children who are stressed, who experience the loss of a loved one, or who have attentional, learning, conduct, or anxiety disorders.

Some researchers have argued that the shifting economic structure of contemporary life has in turn led to profound changes in the organization of family life and that these changes have put the children in these families at far greater risk for depression. The economic demands on families have meant that mobility is rewarded. Furthermore, the demand that both parents work means that that there is less time for family life. The creation of suburbs and the demand for mobility has frequently led to a separation from the extended family and the emotional support that this family can provide.

What Triggers Depression in Children and Teens?

The reasons for depression can vary from child to child. Often, depression results from a combination of factors. Significant events, such as the death of a loved one, parents' divorce, moving away from home, or breaking up with a girlfriend or boyfriend, can trigger symptoms of depression. Neglect, physical, emotional, and sexual abuse, and bullying can also trigger significant depression in children. The effects of trauma in particular can become particularly stressful as a child ages. This is because, as a young child, the victim did not have the life context to process these painful experiences. This stress is aggravated when the adults in their life deny or dismiss that the abuse ever happened. Another trigger can be the hormonal and physical changes that occur during puberty that are often associated with moodiness and rapidly shifting emotions.

Adolescents and Antidepressant Medications: Just the Facts

When Caroline's mother found the journal of her fourteen-year-old daughter, she read what she considered to be part of the normal experiences of a typical honor-roll student. Caroline talked about her drive to keep her grades up, and she noted how happy her parents and her teachers appeared to be with her academic success. Still, as ninth grade wore on, this drive to achieve developed into a severe anxiety disorder, which eventually led the family to seek professional help. She was started on antidepressants to treat the anxiety, and she started therapy to get to the root cause of her worries. Eight months later, her mother found Caroline hanging in her closet. Only hours earlier, she had been out with friends having pizza. Caroline did not leave a note, and her mother felt that the antidepressant medication had led to Caroline's suicide. Advocates for the use of antidepressants point out that the teen suicide rate increased from 5.9 to 11.1 per 100,000 between 1970 and 1994 but declined to 7.4 per 100,000 in 2002, just when the drugs were increasingly being prescribed for children.

Parents often worry about using antidepressant medications in adolescents. The Food and Drug Administration (FDA) looked at this question and recommended that parents weigh the risks versus benefits of their decision, taking the following factors into account.

Risk of Injury to Self or Suicide. It is important to recognize that children or teenagers with depression sometimes think about suicide. They may even try to kill themselves, and, as noted, suicide is a leading cause of death in this group. Antidepressants may increase suicidal thoughts or actions in some children and teens.

The FDA has reported on the combined results of twenty-four different smaller studies of children and teenagers who took either placebo or antidepressants for one to four months. Although no one committed suicide in these studies, some young patients became suicidal. On placebo, 2 of every 100 became suicidal. On the antidepressants, 4 of every 100 young patients became suicidal. The research shows that teens on antidepressants are twice as likely to have suicidal thoughts on antidepressants as on sugar pills.

How to Prevent Self-Injury or Suicide. Patients, parents, teachers, therapists, and doctors should pay close attention to kids on antidepressants and watch for sudden changes in their moods or behaviors. Especially during the early stages of antidepressant use or during dose increases, their prescribing doctors and therapists should monitor teens more regularly.

What to Watch for in Children or Teens Taking Antidepressants. The following would indicate the need for immediate attention and might indicate that the antidepressant medication is causing adverse psychiatric side effects: new or additional thoughts of suicide; trying to commit suicide; new or worse depression; new or worse anxiety; feeling very agitated or restless; panic attacks; difficulty sleeping (insomnia); new or worse irritability; acting aggressive, being angry or violent; acting on dangerous impulses; and being extremely hyperactive in actions and talking (hypomania or mania).

The Benefits and Risks of Antidepressants. Many parents consider these risks to outweigh the potential benefits of these medications. However, antidepressants have been shown to be an effective therapy for depression. Untreated depression can lead to suicide. In some people, treatment with an antidepressant causes suicidal thinking or actions or makes them worse. Deciding what to do involves the psychiatrist or prescribing doctor, the patient, and the patient's parents or guardians reviewing all treatment choices, including the use of antidepressants.

Of all antidepressants, only fluoxetine (brand name Prozac) has been FDA approved to treat pediatric depression. Depression in the young has its own presentation, and treatment of the depression can pose its own risks. The elderly face their own set of challenges when it comes to depression and its treatment.

Depression in the Elderly: The Other End of the Spectrum

Marianne was a seventy-five-year-old retired schoolteacher, who was widowed five years ago when her husband of forty years died of lung cancer. Her three children had successful marriages and careers, and, although none lived nearby, they kept in regular contact with her.

One winter day, she slipped and fell on a patch of ice as she got out of her car and was rushed to the hospital for emergency surgery to replace a broken hip. Her children took time off to help her around the house after her discharge from the hospital, and, as she improved, they turned over these duties to a visiting occupational therapist for continued rehabilitation and a home health aid who helped with groceries and small errands.

Marianne noticed that, soon after her children left, her mood worsened, and, with that, she gradually began to lose weight as her appetite decreased. She felt increasingly tired and told her health aid that she no longer wanted to go to the water acrobics classes at the physical rehabilitation center. She made many excuses to dissuade her bridge-playing friends from visiting for their regular card game.

Her oldest son noted that his mother developed an increasingly negative outlook, often referring to herself as a "burden on my children" and "a useless old woman." With ongoing neglect of her self-care and increasing isolation, and just five months after her accident, she reluctantly agreed to move to an assisted-living facility. There, she began to complain about pain from her hip and walked less and then insisted that she needed assistance to walk and developed a fear of falling.

The facility's consultant psychiatrist diagnosed Marianne as having a major depression. He attempted to treat the depression, but Marianne could not tolerate the side effects of any of the prescribed medications. She was eventually referred to a geriatric psychiatrist who recommended a hospitalization for ECT.

Following a four-week hospitalization and ten ECT treatments, Marianne was discharged back to her assisted-living apartment at the retirement village. Her mood improved noticeably in the weeks following the ECT, and she returned to a more regular schedule of daily walking and weekly bridge games and regular contact with her family.

Symptoms of Depression in the Elderly

A common misconception is that depression is a normal part of aging. Clinical depression is not normal at any age and should always be considered a medical condition that can and should be treated. Untreated depression in the elderly is more likely to lead to suicide than in any other age group. Every day in the United States, seventeen adults over the age of sixty-five commit suicide, the highest suicide rate of any age group. Unlike younger people, those for whom an attempted suicide is seen more as a "cry for help," elderly people who attempt suicide usually succeed. Another sobering statistic is that depression in the elderly affects about six million Americans, but only 10 percent receive treatment. Another significant finding is that 20–25 percent of the elderly in nursing homes are clinically depressed.

It is not unusual for elderly people to experience sadness, social isolation, and loneliness, but clinical depression is characterized by a persistent low mood that does not lift. It interferes significantly with ordinary life functions or activities and can lead to suicide. Because some of these symptoms are similar to those caused by other conditions, such as dementia, which is also more common in the elderly, it is important that a geriatric psychiatrist be consulted for an evaluation. It is also helpful to be aware of the range of symptoms described below and not to rely on sadness alone as an indication of depression. Research has shown that many elderly do not think of themselves as sad, even when there are many of the classic symptoms of depression. Although many of these symptoms are similar to those in the general adult population, depression in the elderly should also be considered when they complain of persistent, vague, or unexplained physical complaints, have memory problems and difficulty in concentrating, lack of playfulness and an inability to laugh, and prolonged grief in the context of the loss of a loved one, particularly if this grief is associated with suicidality. Another challenge for the clinician is to not miss the depression because of a coexisting medical condition that can have similar symptoms. Symptoms are sometimes ignored or considered to be part of Parkinson's disease, Alzheimer's disease, strokes, or heart disease, and, as such, the depression is left undiagnosed.

What Causes Depression in the Elderly?

Although the same biological causes lead to depression in the elderly, they are at greater risk because of their increasing exposure to the following. They are more likely to suffer from the frustration of memory loss and decreasing thinking abilities. They are more likely to have required surgeries that lead to changes in body image, such as amputation as a consequence of diabetes or cancer. They are more likely to suffer from chronic medical illnesses associated with depression such as heart disease and Parkinson's disease. Sometimes the medications used to treat these conditions can lead to depression as a side effect. They begin to consider their own death and mortality, especially as they see their own elderly friends pass away. Retirement sometimes brings an unwelcome slowing down and sense of lost purpose. Poor nutrition can lead to vitamin and mineral deficiencies, which are also associated with depression. Another finding is that people who develop their first depression in old age are likely to have poor circulation, which in turn can lead to reduced blood flow to the brain, which can affect the functioning of brain chemicals such as serotonin.

Considerations in Treating Depression in the Elderly

Treating depression in the elderly can be difficult thanks to cultural stereotypes and attitudes among an older generation that often views depression as a character weakness and not the disease it actually is. Those born after the Great Depression and who experienced World War II often feel as if they simply need to "toughen up" and feel that they are a burden if they ask for help. They might feel that they are too old to get help or that the depression will go away by itself. Even when they consider getting help, they often find that their physical and social isolation makes it hard to know to whom to turn.

Despite these challenges, it is essential that depression be treated for more than the depression itself, because research has shown that depression substantially increases the likelihood of death from physical illnesses. Untreated depression can interfere with a person's ability to follow the necessary treatment regimen or to participate in a rehabilitation program. From a healthcare cost perspective, costs of elderly people with significant symptoms of depression are roughly 50 percent higher than those of nondepressed seniors.

If healthcare workers are aware of the possibility and recognize the symptoms in an older person, the depression is generally easily treated. Medication must be considered as a treatment option, and, with today's newer generation of antidepressant drugs, the side effects of the older classes of drugs can be avoided. Doctors usually start these drugs at lower than recommended dosing to further reduce the risk of side effects. This in part is one reason why evidence shows that antidepressants take longer to start working in the elderly than in younger populations. Another consideration, however, is that the elderly are more likely to have coexisting medical conditions, and, when taken together, some antidepressant drugs can interact with other drugs in adverse ways. It is important that each of the treating doctors be aware of all the different medications and dosages of medication that their patient is taking.

Because of the medication-related concerns in the elderly, psychotherapy should always be considered. This is supported by research findings that brief psychotherapy, which is a talk therapy that helps a person in day-to-day relationships or in learning to counter the distorted negative thinking of depression, is effective in reducing symptoms in short-term depression in older persons who are medically ill. Psychotherapy is also useful in older patients who cannot or will not take medication.

Many communities have established elder centers that cater to providing more than just companionship and offer enriching activities such as continuing education and volunteer opportunities. It is also the case that many older people find their way to a religious congregation, which can provide comfort as they increasingly contemplate their own mortality.

Having considered what depression looks like, who gets it, and how race, age, and gender affect its presentation, an important question remains: why do people get depression? In the next chapter, we consider this question and look at the various causes of depression.

3

Causes of Depression

Exactly what causes depression is not understood. Certainly no specific cause for depression has been identified, but a number of factors are involved. This is probably best illustrated by giving a case example and examining these factors. Larry was an obese fifty-seven-year-old who had worked as a bartender for past thirteen years. Prior to that, he had worked in a steel mill as an administrator for more than twenty years, a job he found soon after graduating from high school. He had been married for thirty years and had three sons who are in good health. He smoked more than a pack of cigarettes per day for the past forty years. As a child, Larry had recurrent rheumatic fever that had resulted in heart complications. He had to have his heart valves replaced in his early forties but then developed heart failure a few years later. This in turn led to low blood flow to his brain with ensuing brain damage. Because of his obesity, he also developed diabetes, arthritis in his knees, sleep apnea, and high blood pressure. He had an unhappy childhood with a father who was abusive and an alcoholic and a mother who herself was chronically ill. Both his mother and his sister were being treated for clinical depression. Furthermore, his wife suffered from hypertension and had recently lost her sales job of more than twenty years.

The Ancients would have insisted that it was an imbalance in Larry's humors that flowed through his body that led to depression. Modern science no longer regards the humoral theory as valid, but many clinicians and scientists talk of there being a "chemical imbalance" in the brain, and many of the contemporary environmental "causes" were recognized by our ancestral physicians.

Larry's case is typical of a patient with chronic medical illnesses developing depression. The contributing factors can be divided into those that made Larry vulnerable to depression, those that triggered the actual depression, and those that perpetuated the depression. In this case, Larry's vulnerability factors included his genetic risk because his mother suffered from depression, his chronic medical illness as a child, and his unavailable abusive and alcoholic father.

The cause of depression is complex. Multiple genes interacting with one another and with the physical and social environment probably influence the development of the illness. Furthermore, many of the genes involved likely require specific environmental circumstances for depression to occur. Whereas no singular cause for depression has been discovered, research shows that the following three broad factors play a role.

FACTOR 1: GENES AND DEPRESSION

Starting from the earliest moment of conception, the first factor to consider is heredity. The tendency to develop depression may be inherited. Looking at all the research studies, it appears that depression is somewhere between 35–70 percent inherited. Every one of these studies noted, however, that the development of depression in people with strong family histories of depression, however likely, involved an interaction of several genes with environmental events.

Twin Studies

Much of what we know about the genetic influence of clinical depression is based on research that has been done with identical twins. Studies on identical twins are useful in research because identical twins have the identical genetic code. In depression studies, research shows that, when one identical twin becomes depressed, the other will also develop depression approximately 76 percent of the time. Even when identical twins are raised apart from each other, that is in different environments, if one develops a depression, the other one will develop depression 67 percent of the time. These findings imply a very strong genetic influence. However, if the issue were purely genetic, then if one twin suffered from depression their identical twin would suffer from depression 100 percent of the time. Other factors influence a person's vulnerability to depression. Fraternal twins are twins that do not have identical genetic codes. Like any siblings, fraternal twins share about 50 percent of the genetic codes. When research is done on fraternal twins, the result is that, when one fraternal twin becomes depressed, the other also develops depression about 19 percent of the time. This is a higher rate of depression when compared with overall rates for the general public but also clearly not as high as for identical twins.

What are the elements that are inherited? Part of the problem in answering this question is that making sense of the genetic map for depression is complicated by the fact that the complex interactions between genes and the environment are neither adequately assessed nor understood. For instance, drug and alcohol abuse are influenced by many genetic factors, such as a person's metabolism, individual variations in responses to the drugs and alcohol, personality types, other physical illnesses, etc. Furthermore, multiple environmental factors that promote or deter excessive drug and alcohol consumption, such as peer relationships, drug and alcohol availability, financial status, employment status, etc., are important. Making sense of the interactions of the environmental and genetic factors is very complicated.

Depression and drug and alcohol abuse have genetic and environmental components that interact and are often diagnosed as co-occurring disorders. Neurogenetic studies have suggested that disruptions in serotonin function are sometimes shared by these disorders. The same case of shared pathology and shared environmental problems could be made for thousands of other illnesses interacting with depression.

These are complex interactions, but there are some obvious genetic influences that are simpler to understand. For instance, as we saw in Chapter 2, research shows that people with depression have lower levels of the brain chemicals serotonin and norepinephrine. People with depression might inherit genes that lead to the production of lower levels of serotonin. In fact, research has found such genes.

Depression and the Attack of the Mutant Genes

In 2004, Dr. Marc Caron, Ph.D., and his colleagues at Duke University (Zhang et al. 2004) announced that they had discovered a variation of the gene that makes serotonin in mice. This particular variation of the serotonin gene led to a 50–70 percent reduction in serotonin production. This suggested that such a variant gene might also exist in humans and might be involved in mood and anxiety disorders. In 2005, the same researchers published that they found the same gene in humans and discovered that this mutant gene was found to be ten times more prevalent in depressed patients than in subjects who were not depressed. It was carried by nine of eighty-seven (10 percent) depressed patients, three of 219 (1.3 percent) healthy controls, and none of sixty bipolar disorder patients. Interestingly, the three control-group carriers also had family histories of psychiatric problems and experienced mild depression and anxiety symptoms, although they did not formally meet criteria for depression.

The researchers also found that patients with the mutation failed to respond well to the selective-serotonin reuptake inhibitor (SSRI) medications, which increase the amount of serotonin in the brain. They concluded that the presence of the mutant gene could underlie a treatment-resistant subtype of the illness.

Drawing the Short Gene

In another study, researchers found an interesting interplay between genes and environment (Caspi et al. 2003). They looked at the serotonin transporter gene. This gene regulates levels of serotonin in the brain. The researchers found that individuals who have a particular variation in the serotonin transporter gene were more likely to develop depression after exposure to stress. As with all genes, everyone carries two copies of the transporter gene. One copy is inherited from the mother and the other from the father. The transporter comes in one of two variations, either a short or long variant. This allows for three possible combinations: people can carry two copies of the short variant, two copies of the long variant, or one copy of each. Whereas both the short form and the long form are common in humans, nearly two-thirds of the population carries at least one copy of the short variation. It turns out that people who carry at least one copy of the short variation of the transporter gene are more vulnerable to depression after they experience a stressful event, whereas people with two copies of the long variation appear to be protected from depression.

In the study, they looked at 847 adults living in New Zealand, assessed what type of gene they had, evaluated any signs of depression within the previous year, and recorded their stressful life events over a five-year period. Life events included unemployment, financial problems, homelessness, physical illness, abuse, and intimate relationship breakups. Thirty-three percent of the people who experienced four or more stressful life events and had at least one copy of short variant developed depression compared with 17 percent of those carrying two copies of the long variant. It appears that having the short variation of the gene is a risk factor for developing depression in those people who experience significantly stressful life events.

As research continues to unravel the secrets of the DNA code, many other such inherited genetic factors will be discovered.

FACTOR 2: MEDICAL CONDITIONS CAUSING DEPRESSION

The triggering factors for Larry's depression in adulthood include the severity of his unrelenting and chronic medical problems. These problems can make many patients feel overwhelmed, out of control, and that nothing they do can stop the rapid progression of their illness. For Larry, his heart failure led to brain damage, which in turn led to depression, cognitive deficits, and personality changes. His sleep apnea caused chronic sleep problems, which led to low energy, exhaustion, and depression.

Factors that perpetuated his depression included his functional decline, which led to a decrease in exercise and recreational activities, which had previously been a source of purpose and pleasure. His cognitive decline also perpetuated his depression because this led to increased difficulties in performing his work duties. A final perpetuating factor was the loss of his wife's job, which led to the stress of having to survive on one salary. Her own physical illness made the maintenance of the household gradually more difficult.

People diagnosed with chronic illness have to adjust to the complications and the treatments of the illness itself. For instance, some medications that treat hypertension cause sedation, which aggravates the low energy state of depression. The illness can affect a person's mobility and independence, their self-image, and their relationships. Although it seems clear that a normal response to such a dramatic change in functioning includes despair and sadness, at times the medical condition can cause a clinical depression.

The case of Larry's depression is illustrative of what happens for many people with chronic illness. Depression is one of the most common complications of chronic illness, and chronic illness clearly causes depression in some people. In Greek mythology, Chronos was the god of time who emerged from the early primordial chaos to establish a sense of order. From the word chronos, we get the word chronic, which, when applied to illness, is usually defined as a persistent and lasting condition. The U.S. National Center for Health Statistics defines a chronic condition as one with a duration of three months or longer. It is generally regarded that such chronic illnesses cannot be completely cured.

Any chronic condition can cause or trigger a clinical depression, but the risk increases with the severity of the illness and the level of disruption it has caused to a person's functioning. Chapter 1 shows that, over a lifetime, the risk of getting depression is generally 10–25 percent for women and 5–12 percent for men. However, in people with chronic illness, the risk increases to between 25 and 33 percent. The rate of depression occurring with chronic medical illnesses is as follows: heart attack, 40–65 percent experience depression; coronary artery disease, 18–20 percent; Parkinson's disease, 40–50 percent; multiple sclerosis, 40 percent; stroke, 10–27 percent; cancer, 25 percent; and diabetes, 25 percent. Other chronic conditions commonly triggering depression are as follows: epilepsy, Alzheimer's disease, Huntington's disease, chronic fatigue syndrome, mononucleosis, endocrine disorders, hypothyroidism, hyperthyroidism, Addison's disease, Cushing's disease, prolactinoma, hyperparathyroidism, and infectious diseases such as HIV, syphilis, and Lyme disease.

Chronic infectious diseases often precipitate a depression. The following case is illustrative. John was a forty-nine-year-old male prison inmate infected with HIV and the hepatitis C virus after years of intravenous heroin injection and sharing needles. His HIV and hepatitis C were under control on a combination of antiviral medications, but he complained to the prison psychiatrist that, ever since the death of his girlfriend from complications of AIDS some 4 months earlier, he noted a persistently low mood, feelings of anger "all the time," difficulty in falling asleep and waking up early in the morning, and increasing thoughts of dying. Furthermore, the thought of taking yet another pill affirmed for him his sense that he had lost complete control of his life. His incarceration, chronic infections with repeated medical treatments, and the loss of his girlfriend precipitated a clinical depression. If left untreated, his depression would not only compromise his medical treatments because his lack of self-care would lead to poor medication compliance, but, more seriously, his feelings of hopelessness could lead to suicide.

Symptoms of Depression in People with Chronic Illness

Clinicians, patients, and their family members often overlook the symptoms of depression. It is often assumed that feeling depressed is normal for someone struggling with a serious, chronic illness. Furthermore, symptoms of depression are often masked by the other medical conditions, so for instance difficulty in moving because of arthritis may mask the low energy of depression, and the difficulties of sleep apnea can hide the sleep problems of depression.

Treatment of Depression in People with Chronic Illness

Treatment of depression in people with chronic disease is similar to that offered to other people with depression. It is essential to assess first for the risk of suicide and then to reduce the distress and despair of the depression. To the extent that the medical illness is causing the depression, the medical illness must be treated, and the psychiatrist and physician rating the medical illness need to coordinate their treatment regimens. For instance, because some psychiatric medications are broken down in the liver, it might be ill considered for a psychiatrist to use such a medication in a person with chronic liver illness. Furthermore, the side effects of psychiatric medication might worsen the underlying medical condition; for instance, some antidepressants cause abnormal heartbeats and so using such medications in people with cardiac disorders would be problematic. Research shows that more than 80 percent of people with depression can be treated successfully with medicine, psychotherapy, or a combination of both.

ENVIRONMENTAL CAUSES OF DEPRESSION

Liana was a twenty-year-old woman who lived at home with her verbally abusive parents who would tell her that she was stupid, unable to do anything right, and that no one would ever love her. Her own image of herself was based on the belief that her parent's perspectives were accurate. She presented to the outpatient clinic feeling helpless and that most of the events and decisions in her life were beyond her control. This feeling of helplessness put her at risk for developing clinical depression at some point in her life, but the feeling had been caused by the repeated accusations and judgments of her parents rather than any innate biological problem Liana had.

Environmental causes of depression are considered to be those factors that lie outside of the individual person. They are the factors that are not directly related to brain function, inherited traits from parents, or medical illnesses. Environmental factors leading to depression are the stressful events that happen in the course of a person's life. There are many such potential life events, such as prolonged stress at home or work, the loss of a loved one, the loss of a job or income, trauma, and juggling the demands of home, work, and relationships. It has long been known that such experiences can affect a person's state of mind. Ultimately how a person reacts to these environmental events will influence the development of clinical depression.

The development of depression under these adverse or stressful circumstances is based on what scientists call the theory of "learned helplessness." This theory states that, when a person experiences chronic or repeated stressful life events, they learn to feel helpless. This feeling of helplessness is strengthened when a person believes they have no control over the stressful situation. People who are depressed very often have negative beliefs about their ability to manage aspects of their lives based on perceived failures in the past. Given the multitude of possible external factors, a few of the environmental causes are presented below.

Seeing the Light of Day

Another environmental factor is the amount of light to which a person is exposed. In Chapter 1, we identified seasonal affective disorder (SAD) as a type of depressive disorder. This occurs most frequently in the winter when daylight hours are short. In the dark, the body produces increased levels of melatonin, which is thought to play a major part in the onset of SAD. It also appears that this effect is reversed by exposure to certain types of light, which thereby treats the depression.

Too Much "Girl Talk"

A twenty-four-year-old patient who suffered from depression once told me that she had gone on a four-hour hike with a new friend who began to tell her about all the problems she was having in her life and her worsening relationship with her boyfriend. After a couple of hours, my patient recognized that she wasn't enjoying the hike and said to her walking companion, "Don't you have a friend you could talk to about this stuff?" My patient felt awful when she realized what she had said but also recognized that all this "problems talk" was too much and that her own mood had been affected. Research shows that in fact this is not an unusual finding.

Dr. Amanda Rose, Ph.D. (Rose, Carlson, and Waller 2007) and colleagues at the University of Missouri-Columbia studied 813 adolescent boys and girls and found that what appeared to be normal, healthy and harmless "girl talk" could lead to depression. In their study, the researchers looked at the effects of excessively talking about their problems, a behavior known as "co-rumination," amongst adolescents and their friends. They found that adolescent girls who excessively talked about every aspect of their problems were more likely to show signs of depression and anxiety, but this was not the case for boys. One hypothesis is that girls tend to internalize their problems and blame themselves, and boys tend to externalize and blame others for their problems.

It seems that, although it is emotionally healthy for adolescents to talk about their problems, such talk in excess is like too much of a good thing and ends up leading to emotional distress. An important finding in the study was that one benefit of co-rumination in both girls and boys was that adolescents who did so ended up feeling closer to their friends. The trick is to get this healthy benefit, the closeness to friends, but avoid the unhealthy complication of depression. Ideally, this is done by having a professional therapist address some of the more difficult aspects of whatever problem exists.

Life Experiences

Early life experiences, such as the death of a parent and physical, psychological, or sexual abuse, also increase the likelihood of depression later in life. Social rejection, drug use, and bullying in adolescence contribute to the development of depression. Later life experiences, such as unemployment, financial difficulties, the loss of a partner or other family member, divorce, or domestic violence, can also trigger depression.

An Empty Diet

Omega-3 fatty acids are considered essential fatty acids, which means that they are essential to human health but cannot be manufactured by the body. These fatty acids are important components of nerve cell membranes. They help nerve cells communicate with each other, which is an essential step in maintaining good mental health. The increase in rates of depression in industrialized countries has been linked to a highly refined diet and particularly to dramatically lower levels of omega-3 fatty acids because of intensive farming and livestock rearing methods. Furthermore, countries that have high omega-3 fat consumption have lower rates of depression. Fish and fish oil, as well as flax seed oil, are rich sources of omega-3 fats, and adding these fats to the contemporary Western diet has been shown to reduce depression.

Recreational Drug Use

Whereas some people use drugs and alcohol as self-medication to treat depression, many who abuse drugs and alcohol end up affecting their emotional, psychological, and relational health, in turn causing depression. Some drugs, such as methamphetamine, can seriously affect neurotransmitter and brain function, at times leading to long-lasting or permanent damage. Generally, the longer people abuse the drugs, the more likely they are to suffer from depression.

Prescribed Drug Use

There are a number of common prescription drugs that have side effects that can induce depression. These include some cardiac drugs, sedatives, steroids, stimulants, and antibiotics. In some cases, the underlying medical condition can cause a depression, and this depression is aggravated by the side effects of the drugs used to treat the medical condition.

The cause of depression will always be the interaction between a person's genes, their biology, and their environment. Having an understanding of the factors that trigger or contribute to depression is essential for two main reasons. First, knowing the causes can help researchers and clinicians develop ways to prevent depression as in developing stress reduction programs for people with the short variation of the serotonin transporter gene or developing early substance abuse intervention with young adolescents. Second, and as important, understanding the causes can lead to better treatments, and it is with this in mind that we move onto the topic of treatment in the next chapter.

4

Treatment of Depression

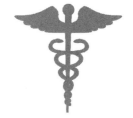

DEVELOPMENTS LEADING TO CONTEMPORARY TREATMENTS OF DEPRESSION

The ancients cured depression through bloodletting, skull drilling, herbs, solar therapy, prayer, and the casting out of demons. The twentieth century produced the science to develop new treatments and the research to validate or debunk the older remedies. An important observation recognized by all treaters was that, although major depression in its most severe form is a devastating and lethal illness, most people who suffer from the condition get better with treatment.

The Early Physical Treatments: Sleep, Shock, and Surgery

"We went through the top of the head, I think she was awake. She had a mild tranquilizer. I made a surgical incision in the brain through the skull. It was near the front. It was on both sides. We just made a small incision, no more than an inch." The instrument Dr. Watts used looked like a butter knife. He swung it up and down to cut brain tissue. "We put an instrument inside," he said. As Dr. Watts cut, Dr. Freeman put questions to Rosemary. For example, he asked her to recite the Lord's Prayer or sing "God Bless America" or count backwards. "We made an estimate on how far to cut based on how she responded." When she began to become incoherent, they stopped.

(James W. Watts, quoted in Kessler 1997, 226)

This was how the neurosurgeon James Watts describes the surgical procedure performed on Rosemary Kennedy in 1941. Rosemary was the older sister of president John F. Kennedy. She was twenty-three years old when she had the lobotomy, which her father Joseph requested to deal with Rosemary's mood swings that her family found difficult to handle, tantrums, rages, and violent behavior. She had physical fights, and at times, some nights, she would be found wandering the streets. She had also developed an excessive interest in sex and her family feared that she would become pregnant. The family said that she showed poor judgment in situations and that she had mild mental retardation, which further justified the brain surgery.

Years later, author Ronald Kessler interviewed Dr. Watts who told the author that, in his opinion, "Rosemary had suffered not from mental retardation but from a form of depression.... It may have been agitated depression, you're agitated, you're shaky. You talk in an agitated way."

Lobotomy and Brain Surgery for Depression and Other Mental Illnesses

Rosemary Kennedy owed her fate to Antonio Moniz, a Portuguese psychiatrist who felt that some forms of mental illness were caused by abnormal brain nerve cell connections where messages would get stuck. This would lead to a loop in which the messages were repeated over and over again, leading to mental disorders. Moniz felt that if, these connections could be found and destroyed, the patients would get better.

In 1935, he tested his theory by injecting alcohol into the frontal lobes of mentally ill patients. After this, he would cut the frontal lobe with a wire, without removing any part of the brain. A year later, he published the results of his first twenty operations on patients who had suffered from anxiety, depression, and schizophrenia and showed remarkably positive results.

His first patient was less paranoid and agitated than she had been before, although she was also more dull and listless than she had been before. His results lead to the widespread acceptance of this new procedure. In 1949, he was awarded the Nobel Prize in Medicine "for his discovery of the therapeutic value of leucotomy in certain psychoses." More than 20,000 people would go on to have the procedure performed in the United States alone.

In 1949, Rosemary Kennedy, incapacitated by the lobotomy that had markedly worsened her cognitive abilities, was moved to the St. Coletta School in

Jefferson, Wisconsin, a residential institution for people with disabilities. Due to the severity of her mental condition, Rosemary became largely detached from the Kennedy family, except for the visits of her sister Eunice Kennedy Shriver, who later founded the Special Olympics in Rosemary's memory.

Brain surgery to treat depression and other mental illnesses was a product of the twentieth century. Starting in the early 1900s, there was renewed interest in physical treatments for depression, just at the time that Freud's "talking cure" for psychiatric illness was taking off. In 1920, the psychiatrist Jakob Klasi developed sleep therapy in which he used a drug-induced sleep that lasted as long as six days to treat depression and to calm hysterical patients. His hypothesis was that the nervous system was exhausted and needed rest. It may go without saying that this treatment did not work, despite its interest at the time.

Ironically, 2005 brought research into a sleeping therapy for "depression." There is a group of patients who experience, among other symptoms, sleepiness, fatigue, poor motivation, irritability, and difficulty concentrating. Many of these patients are frequently diagnosed with depression and are treated with antidepressants. A fuller history might also have elicited symptoms of memory problems, weight gain, headaches, and job impairment. It appears that many of these patients suffer not from depression but obstructive sleep apnea, which is caused by a blockage of the upper airways during sleep, leading to frequent awakenings. When the airway is blocked, with each episode of airway blockage or "apnea," the brain awakens the person to get them to start breathing again, but, because of this, sleep is terribly disrupted and of very poor quality.

Treatment for these symptoms is not antidepressant medications, despite the similarity to depression, but a treatment called continuous positive airway pressure (CPAP) therapy. CPAP delivers air into the airway through a specially designed mask. Airflow creates enough pressure to keep the airway open, which means that the person does not wake up and their quality of sleep improves dramatically. This in turn frequently resolves "depression" symptoms, effectively leading to a sleeping cure.

Another physical treatment for depression was the so-called "carbon dioxide therapy." In this therapy, the patients were administered a gas solution that had a high concentration of carbon dioxide, which was thought to have a dual antidepressant effect. First, it was thought to move the person deeply into their psyche, which would "help them find significant issues." Second, it made the depressed patients hyperventilate, which appeared to boost their energy levels.

In the late 1930s and early 1940s, there was a battle between two very different perspectives in psychiatry. One the one hand, there were psychiatrists such as Bernard Sachs, who wrote an article *Present Day Trends in Neuro-Psychiatric Research,* in which he reviewed all the chemical, pharmacologic, and electric shock therapy of the time and urged neuropsychiatrists to continue the research. Psychoanalytically trained psychiatrists such as Gregory Zilboorg represented the other side of the argument. He felt that some of the "physical therapies" such as shock therapy were "abhorrent." He appeared to insist that the cures had to be psychological and that the chance cure of a patient using a "physical cure" had to have a psychological explanation.

One of the new cures was metrazol convulsive treatment, which became popular in the 1930s. Metrazol is a chemical that induces a state of such fear that it leads to convulsions. Because it was so effective, it was widely used to treat depression. Study after study showed the remarkable effect of metrazol on depression. In a case report by Grotjahn, a fifty-four-year-old female patient treated on metrazol reported that, "I hated everything. I even hated the door, the rug under the table. During the metrazol treatments I put myself in your hands. It was like being reborn. The hate left me. I did not give up depression; it just disappeared. I was only watching. The metrazol took the depression out of my hands."

Researchers at the time reported that depressions that had lasted for years went into remission in weeks. Similarly, when American psychiatrist Abram Bennett first used metrazol convulsive shock therapy on patients, he recognized the marked improvement in his patients and in 1938 wrote up a case report of nine patients who had improved on the therapy. In the paper, he wrote, "We cannot explain the mechanism of recovery in these patients but it is physiological in these cases, not psychological."

However, metrazol had its problems. Most significantly, the convulsions caused by the drug were so severe that they caused spine fractures in nearly half of the patients. The search for better cures continued.

The First Drugs

Drugs and medicines have always been a part of the treatment of various conditions. Recorded history is filled with accounts of drugs that altered the mind. Alcohol, for instance, has been widely used and abused and was a problem among ancient Greeks and Romans. There are records of cannabis and opium use in the ancient Middle East. Early in the Middle Ages, Arab traders introduced the use of the opium poppy to India and China. In China, opium was used primarily as a medicine. In India, it became a widespread addiction of the rich, and there are also reports of soldiers using it to enhance their battle spirit. By the seventeeth century, coffee was considered as healthful and therapeutic and was even praised as a substitute for the evil that was alcohol.

An important milestone in the development of medication to treat depression occurred in 1859 when Dr. Pablo Mantegazzo isolated cocaine from the coca leaf and wrote about its wonderful powers to combat fatigue, depression, and impotence. Vin Mariani, a wine mixed with coca, became a major success, and Pope Leo XIII awarded its developer a gold medal for being a benefactor of mankind. Cocaine became a popular drug and became one of the key ingredients in a popular tonic known as Coca-Cola. Until 1903, "Coke" contained 60 milligrams of cocaine per eight ounce serving!

Amphetamine became the first major synthetic drug and was used as a stimulant to treat depression and boost the energy levels of soldiers during World War II. During the 1950s, legally manufactured tablets of both dextroamphetamine (Dexedrine) and methamphetamine (Methedrine) became readily available and were used as stimulants and without medical prescription by college students for better grades, truck drivers to stay awake, and athletes to enhance performance. They were being used as a cure-all for everything from weight control to treating depression.

Despite the concerns of abuse, the promise of an effective pill to treat or even cure depression presented patients with hope and pharmaceutical companies the opportunity for vast riches.

THE PHARMACEUTICAL AGE: BETTER LIVING THROUGH MEDICATION

When Mike Wallace, the CBS TV personality, best known as a correspondent on *60 Minutes*, developed a clinical depression, he attributed his recovery to treatment thus: "Talk ... psychotherapy with that antidepressant medication, Ludiomil. And then, after my 75th birthday, Zoloft, the new selective-serotonin reuptake inhibitor (SSRI) antidepressant had been developed. My psychiatrist prescribed it, played around with the dose to get it right. When he did, that helped a lot."

Medications developed especially to treat depression were first introduced in the 1950s and 1960s. They belonged to a class of medications known as the monoamine oxidase inhibitors (MAOIs) and the tricyclic antidepressants (TCAs). Soon after that, an explosion in the understanding of brain chemistry, and in particular as it pertained to depression, brought with it the development of the SSRIs and the serotonin and norepinephrine reuptake inhibitors (SNRIs) and other medications that are a class onto themselves.

The serotonin and norepinephrine chemicals are the most studied to date, and most modern drug treatments for depression target these chemicals. The most important finding is that people with depression have low levels of serotonin and norepinephrine, and medications that increase these chemicals have been found to be highly effective antidepressants.

When Amy Tan, author of *The Joy Luck Club*, was asked about the effects of her medication treatment for depression, she said, "I take Zoloft. I don't think it's made me a Pollyanna. I can still get angry and upset, but I don't fall into the abyss. I'm grateful that I have some traction now. It doesn't change essentially who you are, but it fixes things just the way insulin does for people with diabetes."

MAOIs

The first class of drugs discovered was known as the MAOIs. They work by inactivating the enzyme monoamine oxidase, which in the brain breaks down serotonin, norepinephrine, and dopamine. By inactivating this enzyme, these chemicals are not broken down, so effectively, their levels increase. They are very effective drugs as antidepressants. The MAOIs include the drugs phenelzine, isocarboxazid, and tranylcypromine sulfate. These are the scientific names of the drugs, and generally drug manufacturers give the drugs easier sounding and more memorable names!

One major problem with the MAOIs is that monoamine oxidase also breaks down the amino acid tyramine. Tyramine is a naturally occurring substance formed from the breakdown of proteins in certain foods, particularly as those foods age. Foods such as aged cheeses, red wines, some cured meats, yeast extract, sauerkraut, draft beer, and fermented soybean products (such as soy sauce) have the highest levels of tyramine. High levels of tyramine can cause a dangerous increase in blood pressure and lead to stroke or terrible headaches and migraines. It is therefore important to avoid foods that are rich in tyramine while taking this class of drugs. This makes these drugs the least safe of the antidepressants. Suicidal patients have been known to have a large meal of aged cheeses and meats with red wine and then take an overdose of MAOIs.

Another major problem is that, because these drugs can linger in the body for up to two weeks, if the MAOI is discontinued, the person would have to wait two weeks before being started on another antidepressant. This is because the new drugs would, for example, increase the level of serotonin, and the MAOI that was left in the body would prevent any of the serotonin from braking down. This in turn would lead to unnaturally high levels of serotonin. When there is too much serotonin floating in the brain, it can lead to a condition known as the serotonin syndrome, which is as ominous as it sounds.

Serotonin syndrome is a rare but potentially life-threatening adverse drug reaction that results from intentional self-poisoning, therapeutic drug use, or inadvertent interactions between drugs. The symptoms usually occur quickly and vary from mild symptoms with a rapid heart rate, excess sweating, and shivering, to moderate symptoms that would include high blood pressure and a high temperature, to severe symptoms including shock, delirium, muscle stiffness, temperature above 105.98°F, kidney failure, and eventually death.

Because of these restrictions and the availability of other drugs, the MAOIs are rarely used today, although they are used when the food restrictions are not an issue, or sometimes in a compliant patient when no other medication has worked.

TCAs

The tricyclic antidepressants are a class of drugs that work by preventing the reuptake or repackaging of the neurotransmitters norepinephrine, dopamine, or serotonin by nerve cells. The neurotransmitter theory of depression is that these "chemicals" are low in the brain. Generally, after a neurotransmitter has been released by a nerve cell, it is either broken down or taken back into the nerve cell. The purpose of taking the neurotransmitter back into the cell is so that it can be repackaged and then used again. This process is known as reuptake. By preventing or blocking the reuptake, more of the chemical is available in the brain, and thus available to counter depression caused by low levels of the chemical. Some of the TCAs are amitriptyline, nortriptyline, desipramine, and imipramine. Again, as with the MAOIs, these are given trade names by their manufacturers.

Although this class of medications works very well for depression, like the MAOIs, they are seldom used today as a first choice for treating depression. This again has to do with potential side effects. The problem is that they can cause bladder problems, constipation, a dry mouth, sexual problems, blurred vision, dizziness, drowsiness, and unwanted weight changes, but the most serious side effect is that they can cause the heart to have abnormal beats and rhythms. When taken in overdose, they can quickly lead to death from heart arrest.

SSRIs

Because of the side effects of the other two drug classes, researchers continued to look for drugs that kept the benefits but eliminated some of the more troublesome and potentially lethal side effects. The SSRIs are the most commonly prescribed class of antidepressants. They work by blocking the reuptake of serotonin from the synapse back into the nerve, thereby increasing the serotonin that is available in the synapse. The SSRIs include the medications fluoxetine (better known as Prozac), sertraline (better known as Zoloft), paroxetine (better known as Paxil), fluvoxamine (better known as Luvox), citalopram (better known as Celexa), and escitalopram (better known as Lexapro). SSRIs are the most effective treatment for premenstrual dysphoric disorder in women, although they may cause a significant worsening of libido. SSRIs do not cause serious birth defects and are considered acceptable for pregnant women.

As sales of SSRIs began to skyrocket, psychiatrists, and in particular child and adolescent psychiatrists, began to notice that children taking these medications especially at adult doses appeared to be becoming increasingly suicidal. The FDA then issued this general warning:

> Antidepressant medications are used to treat a variety of conditions, including depression and other mental/mood disorders. These medications can help prevent suicidal thoughts/attempts and provide other important benefits. However, studies have shown that a small number of people (especially children/teenagers) who take antidepressants for any condition may experience worsening depression, other mental/mood symptoms, or suicidal thoughts/attempts. Therefore, it is very important to talk with the doctor about the risks and benefits of antidepressant medication (especially for children/teenagers), even if treatment is not for a mental/mood condition.

They further required the makers of antidepressants to include this serious side-effect warning (known as a black-box warning) with its marketing materials:

> Antidepressants increase the risk of suicidal thinking and behavior (suicidality) in children and adolescents with MDD and other psychiatric disorders. Anyone considering the use of an antidepressant in a child or adolescent for any clinical use must balance the risk of increased suicidality with the clinical need. Patients who are started on therapy should be observed closely for clinical worsening, suicidality, or unusual changes in behavior. Families and caregivers should be advised to closely observe the patient and to communicate with the prescriber. A statement regarding whether the particular drug is approved for any pediatric indication(s) and, if so, which one(s).

The warning was well advised but perhaps not always well heeded.

Jeff Weise was a sixteen-year-old adolescent living on Red Lake Indian Reservation, a place he detested. In a blog posting, he wrote that people "choose alcohol over friendship" and women neglect "their own flesh and blood" for relationships with men, and he could not escape "the grave I'm continually digging for myself." His earlier life had been no happier, and depression and drug use ran in his family. When he was eight, his father committed suicide on the reservation after a standoff with police. About four months later, his mother suffered severe brain damage in an alcohol-related car accident. Before her accident, his alcoholic mother used to lock him out of her house or her boyfriend would lock him in a closet and made him kneel for hours in a corner. Again, his blog reflected his misery and depression. "I should've taken the razor blade express last time around.... Well, whatever, man. Maybe they've got another shuttle comin' around soon?" For the depression, he had been prescribed Prozac, and, as the depression persisted, the dose was gradually increased from 20 to 60 milligrams per day.

With his loathing of reservation life and burdened by his father's suicide and his mother's abuse, on March 21, 2005, he joined the ranks of America's schoolhouse killers by murdering nine people, his grandfather, his grandfather's female companion, a school guard, a teacher, and five schoolmates, before killing himself.

His aunt told the *New York Times* that she wondered whether the increase in the Prozac had triggered the boy's final rage: "They kept upping the dose for him and by the end, he was taking three of the 20 milligram pills a day. I can't help but think it was too much, that it must have set him off."

Prozac is a medication frequently (and effectively) used in child psychiatry. Jeff Weise's story is a cautionary one, that both (1) medication cannot address the environmental misery of a person's existence and (2) nor should medications like Prozac be automatically increased, especially in adolescents, when they do not appear to be working.

SNRIs

These are the second-most popular antidepressants worldwide. These medications block the reuptake of both serotonin and norepinephrine from the synapse into the nerve, thereby increasing the amounts of these chemicals. The SNRIs are medications such as venlafaxine (Effexor) and duloxetine (Cymbalta). The side effects of these medications are similar to those of the SSRIs, and the ones most frequently encountered are nausea, nervousness, insomnia, diarrhea, rash, agitation, or sexual side effects, such as problems with arousal or orgasm.

Norepinephrine-Dopamine Reuptake Inhibitor

The only norepinephrine-dopamine reuptake inhibitor approved by the FDA is bupropion (Wellbutrin). It is a popular and regularly used antidepressant that acts by blocking the reuptake of dopamine and norepinephrine, again thereby increasing the amounts of these chemicals in the brain. It has been shown to work well in ADHD and nicotine addiction and can help people quit smoking. Some of the downsides to the drug are that, at high doses, it can cause seizures in some people. It can also cause high blood pressure in others. Because high blood pressure is also a side effect of nicotine supplements frequently used by people trying to quit smoking, using both bupropion and nicotine supplements can cause a dangerous elevation in blood pressure. Other common side effects are restlessness, insomnia, headache, tremor, agitation, confusion, rapid heartbeat, dizziness, nausea, constipation, menstrual complaints, and rash.

Noradrenergic and Specific Serotonergic Antidepressant

Mirtazapine (Remeron) is an antidepressant with a tetracyclic chemical structure. It works differently from the other classes of antidepressants because it targets specific serotonin and norepinephrine receptors in the brain, thus indirectly increasing the activity of several brain circuits. Because of its unique pharmacologic profile, it does not cause much in the way of low blood pressure or some of the sexual side effects seen in the other drugs. It can, however, cause drowsiness, increased appetite, and weight gain and at times visual hallucinations if taken in the morning rather than at night.

An Adequate Antidepressant Trial

There are a growing number of antidepressants available for the treatment of depression, and there are times when an antidepressant does not appear to work or gives severe side effects to the patient taking the drug. The prescribing doctor then has to decide whether to continue the medication, increase or decrease the does, or switch medication altogether.

To say that an antidepressant has not worked, a patient has to have been on an adequate trial of the medication. Generally, this is defined as a therapeutic dose of the medication and for a sufficient period of time to achieve a clinical benefit that may require four to six weeks or more.

Unfortunately, a significant number of patients do not stick to their treatment plan. When this happens, it is known as noncompliance when the patient does not take the medication and partial compliance when they do some of the time. Some of the reasons for noncompliance are side effects, drugs that require dosing more than once a day, the use of multiple drugs, feeling better and thinking that they no longer need the drug, or the feeling that the medication is just not going to help. It is also the case that many times patients who stop taking their medication don't inform their prescribing doctor that they have stopped. One common side effect is a reduction in sexual desire, and many patients are embarrassed to talk to their clinicians about this.

To address the premature cessation of medication, clinicians do well in educating their patients about the potential side effects, including sexual side effects, how long the drug will take to work, the dangers of abruptly stopping the medication trial, and the options for what to do if the drug trial fails.

In a 60 *Minutes* interview on CBS, the comedian Jim Carrey said the following:

> I was on Prozac for a long time. It may have helped me out of a jam for a little bit, but people stay on it forever. I had to get off at a certain point because I realized that, you know, everything's just OK. There are peaks, there are valleys. But they're all kind of carved and smoothed out, and it feels like a low level of despair you live in. Where you're not getting any answers, but you're living OK. And you can smile at the office. You know? But it's a low level of despair. You know?

It is not uncommon for people to stop taking their antidepressant medication when they feel their symptoms have improved. Others stop their antidepressant medication because of bothersome side effects despite their mood being better. Although it may seem reasonable to stop taking the medication, the problem is that at least 50 percent of the time the symptoms of depression come back. Certainly any such decision is best made in conjunction with a treating psychiatrist.

Using Drugs in Combination to Treat Depression

Psychiatrists sometimes combine the antidepressants mentioned above either with each other in combination to treat depression or with medications that are not antidepressants themselves. Combining antidepressants with other drugs to get a more robust effect is known as "augmentation." Other medications used in augmentation include the atypical antipsychotic agents, thyroid hormones, the stimulant class of medications, lithium, antianxiety medications, mood-stabilizing medications, and rarely natural remedies that have not been approved by the FDA for the treatment of depression.

Antidepressant drugs have clearly revolutionized the treatment of depression, but almost all studies show that it is the combination of medication and talk therapy that provides the best outcomes for people suffering with depression.

PSYCHOTHERAPY: THE POWER OF TALK

Critics of medication therapy have argued that antidepressant medication only removes the symptoms of depression, but doesn't treat the patient's underlying distorted and destructive attitudes. These attitudes, they argue, can only be addressed in psychotherapy.

Psychotherapy can be broadly defined as a therapy in which the treatment includes that a patient talk with a psychiatrist, psychologist, social worker, or licensed counselor about a mental health condition such as depression. Studies have shown that psychotherapy can be effective in treating mild and moderate forms of depression and can be combined with drug therapy to treat all degrees of depression.

Psychotherapies can be divided into three general categories: individual therapy, couples and family therapy, and group therapy. Typically, the individual therapies are used to treat depression, although occasionally group therapy is prescribed. Family and couples therapy is not generally used as the primary modality for treating depression and is included here for the sake of completeness. Here the categories are described in more detail and as they pertain to the treatment of depression.

Individual Therapies

Interpersonal Therapy

Although depression may not be caused by interpersonal events, it usually has an interpersonal component. The interpersonal theory is that depression can lead to feelings of wanting to isolate or be alone, of not knowing what to say and of feeling uninteresting and wretched. A common finding in people who suffer from depression is a lack of satisfaction in the various relationships in their life. This lack of satisfaction is experienced not only by the sufferer, but also by the others in their life. Family, work, and other social relationships are impacted as the weight of the depression causes a reduction in the energy and desire to sustain these relationships successfully. With ongoing isolation and decreased social interactions the person suffering from depression becomes less assertive, less positive, less interactive, showing less eye contact and becoming less responsive and communicative in relationships.

Interpersonal therapy (IPT) focuses on the way that a person relates, expresses himself or herself, and communicates with the significant others in his or her life. It has the following goals in the treatment of depression: first, to diagnose depression explicitly; to educate the person about depression, its causes, and the various treatments available for it; next, to identify the interpersonal context of depression and how this can affect the depression; finally, to develop strategies for the person to follow in coping with the depression. IPT is a short-term therapy with normally twenty or fewer sessions per therapy. Because of this, the therapist addresses only one or two of the major problem areas in the patient's current functioning. This is determined in the early sessions, when the therapist and patient agree on which areas would be most helpful in reducing the patient's symptoms. The remaining sessions are then directed at resolving these agreed-upon problem areas. Research shows that the targeted approach of IPT can lead to rapid improvement for some patients, with problems ranging from mild situational depression to severe depression. The following is an example of IPT for depression.

Victor was a thirty-year-old man who had lost his job a year ago and had not been able to find work. He subsequently became increasingly depressed. He and his wife were fighting because he wanted a baby, but she felt that they should wait until they were financially more stable. Together with his IPT therapist, he explored the nature of his depression, and Victor recognized that his depression might be related to his job loss and his inability to find a meaningful role for himself.

He also began to appreciate the fact that he was pressuring his wife to become pregnant as a way to give meaning to his life: if he could not be a wage earner, he would be a father. Talking about these feelings with his therapist, Victor began to recognize how much his self-worth was tied into being successfully employed. He realized that he responded to his job loss with anger and shame and that he took his frustrations out on his wife. IPT helped Victor repair his relationship with his wife and understand how losing his role as a breadwinner had made him feel angry and depressed. By repairing his relationship with his wife and recognizing his subsequent shame, he was able to approach subsequent job interviews with less anger and soon thereafter had a meaningful job.

Cognitive Behavioral Therapy

Everything is but what your opinion makes it; and that opinion lies with yourself.

(Marcus Aurelius, *Meditations*)

The cognitive behavioral theory of depression states that a patient's excessive self-rejection and self-criticism leads to major depression. Cognitive behavioral therapy (CBT) targets these negative thoughts to overcome the patient's pessimism and hopelessness. The idea is that, by a person modifying their regular thoughts and behaviors, they will be able to influence their emotions. CBT works on the basic premise that all emotion comes from thoughts. For example, if a person thinks about something scary, they will feel fear. The idea behind the therapy is that people learn to "catch" their thoughts and challenge them so that they can feel differently. Common CBT techniques include keeping a diary of significant events and associated feelings, thoughts, and behaviors. The following vignette clarifies the basics of CBT.

Mark was a successful twenty-eight-year-old salesman who was criticized by his boss for having missed a business opportunity. Mark recognized that, soon after this incident, he started to think that he was useless and that he couldn't "do anything right." The thought continued to repeat and he became increasingly depressed. Embarrassed by his perceived failure, the previously gregarious Mark avoided situations and social activities that involved close contact with friends and coworkers. This led to increasing isolation, further worsening his depression. This led to fewer business leads, thereby reinforcing his idea that he was useless.

In therapy, the cycle of isolation and feeling useless was identified as a self-fulfilling prophecy, and the therapy was aimed at breaking this cycle. This was done by addressing the way that he thought in response to similar situations and by developing more flexible ways to think and respond, including reducing the avoidance of activities. By escaping from the negative thought pattern and reintegrating back into his life, his feelings of depression lifted. As he became more active, Mark became more productive, which in turn further reduced his feelings of depression.

One of the criticisms of CBT is that a depressed patient's pessimistic and negative thoughts are a result of their major depression, not its cause. These critics argue that antidepressant medications have been shown to remove these negative and destructive attitudes. Either way, developing the ability to recognize and change maladaptive patterns of thinking and behavior is a skill that can be used in many different life situations.

Psychoanalytically Oriented Therapy

Psychoanalysis is the form of psychotherapy made famous by Sigmund Freud. It seeks to discover the connections between what he called the "unconscious mind" and current life events. The therapist's goal is to help patients remove whatever is blocking them from examining their unconscious. These blocks were termed "defenses." The psychoanalytic theory of depression is that a person is angry at the world or angry with the close people in their life. They don't take this anger out on the world but rather become self-critical and turn the anger in on themselves. Classically, psychiatrists were taught that depression was "anger turned inwards on the self."

The following vignette is typical of the way a psychoanalyst might see a case of depression. Jones was a thirty-nine-year-old man with a history of bouts

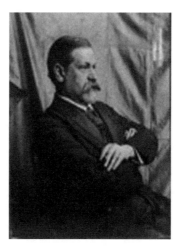

Figure 4.1. Sigmund Freud. *Courtesy Library of Congress, Prints & Photographs Division, LCPP003B-38475.*

of severe depression since his teenage years. His most recent depression had lasted for almost a year, and his symptoms included despair, poor sleep, poor energy, and suicidal thoughts. He was married and had two children. It was after an unsuccessful trial of medication and the sudden death of his mother that he decided to go into psychoanalysis. His analyst noted that, previously, Jones's depression had served to shield him from deeper commitments but that now his ability to work was significantly compromised.

Jones said that, as a child, he had a promising acting career and that his mother pushed him hard and relished in the praise of his abilities. When he was a teenager, his parents divorced. His mother remarried an actor who was thirty-eight, which the analyst noted was close to Jones's present age. His analyst interpreted Jones's depression as a performance, an act to avoid dealing with life. Initially after his mother's death, he was unable to express feelings about her. Jones became angry at his analyst for bringing her up, and it emerged that his history included soiling his pants and being slapped in the face when he confused his lines while being directed by his mother. Through the psychoanalysis, he understood his feelings of being damaged by his mother, enraged at her, and shame at himself. He wished to be strong and available to his own children. The analyst interpreted that the depression served to block the patient from being able to be angry with his mother and explore his own past. By removing this block, he was able to resolve the anger and move on.

Because it may take many years to unblock such defenses, unlike IPT and CBT, psychoanalysis can sometimes take years of therapy. Furthermore, whereas IPT and CBT are usually one hour per week, psychoanalysis is often two to five hours per week. Many have criticized psychoanalysis as taking too long to effect a cure and being too expensive.

Group Therapy

Group therapy is a form of therapy in which a small number of people (usually five to ten) meet together under the leaderships of a psychotherapist with the purpose of helping themselves and one another. Unique to group therapy is that it forces the person to interact in a group, which more closely approximates the group nature of many social interactions. Generally, people are placed with groups of others who suffer from the same condition, a process that allows the person a better chance of feeling validated and understood.

In depression, group therapy addresses feelings of isolation, depression, or anxiety. By encouraging people in the group to talk about their depression, it can help people recognize aspects that they had not considered. Furthermore, because social skills are often compromised in people with depression, the group process allows for the opportunity to practice social interactions.

Family and Couples Therapy

Family therapy has been used synonymously with couples therapy and marriage counseling, although more broadly, family therapy includes family members beyond the immediate couple. It is a form of therapy that works with families and intimate couples to nurture change and development by focusing on the interactions between family members.

Although family therapy is not generally the primary therapy for the treatment of depression, it is prescribed for cases in which either the depression appears to be seriously jeopardizing the person's marriage and family functioning or a person's depression appears to be encouraged and maintained by marital and family interaction patterns. People with mood disorders have a much higher rate of divorce than those without a mood disorder. Nearly 50 percent of spouses report they would not have married their depressed partner or had children had they known that the partner was going to have a mood disorder. Family therapy is an effective approach for educating the family and addressing the effects that a depression has on a family.

Other Forms of Talk Therapy

Religious Psychotherapy and Depression

Prayer tends to be a very individual and private experience. Some therapists have attempted to more formally integrate a person's faith into the therapeutic experience.

Religious psychotherapy (RPT) is an approach to therapy that attempts to recognize and utilize the religious beliefs of clients in treatment for the purposes of reducing mental health difficulties. One review paper summarized the findings of the four scientific studies that looked at whether religious psychotherapy improves anxiety and depression in religious adults (Berry 2002). The researchers found that (1) RPT was as effective as standard treatment for anxiety and depression, (2) the results in each study were statistically significant and appeared to qualify as being clinically significant, and (3) the studies reviewed, although varying in quality, were properly conducted experiments marked by intervention, randomization, and control groups or comparison with standard treatment groups. It is not so much the specific faith or practice, but incorporating a person's religious beliefs into psychotherapy appears to lead to the reduction of distressing symptoms.

Prayer for Depression

When we were children, my devoutly Catholic grandmother used to tell us the stories of the Catholic Saints. Among the stories was the story of St. Dymphna from the seventh century. The story goes that, when Dymphna was fourteen her mother died. Dymphna's father, Damon, a pagan Irish king, is said to have become profoundly depressed, brought on by the grief of the loss of his wife. He wanted to replace his wife with a woman of noble birth and who physically resembled his wife, but, when none could be found, he was advised to marry his daughter. Dymphna fled from her castle to Belgium with an elderly priest. Damon ordered that the priest's head be cut off and then asked his daughter to return to Ireland. When she refused, the king himself decapitated his own daughter. For her faith and willingness to die for her faith, she was made a saint. Specifically, she is the patron saint of families, insanity, and mental illness professionals as well as incest victims, epileptics, runaways, and those suffering from mental illness. All faiths have some form of prayer or contemplation used for depression and other mental anguish. Some examples follow.

Here is a Catholic prayer for depression (prayed to St. Dymphna):

Lord God, who has graciously chosen St. Dymphna to be the patroness of those afflicted with mental and nervous disorders, and has caused her to be an inspiration and a symbol of charity to the thousands who invoke her intercession, grant through the prayers of this pure, youthful martyr, relief and consolation to all who suffer from these disturbances, and especially to those for whom we now pray. (Here mention those for whom you wish to pray.) We beg You to accept and grant the prayers of St. Dymphna on our behalf. Grant to those we have particularly recommended patience in their sufferings and resignation to Your Divine Will. Fill them with hope and, if it is according to Your Divine Plan, bestow upon them the cure they so earnestly desire. Grant this through Christ Our Lord. Amen.

Does prayer help for depression or other mental illnesses? David Hodge, an assistant professor of social work in the College of Human Services at Arizona State University, conducted a very large study on the effects of prayer among people with psychological or medical problems (Hodge 2007). His research looked at seventeen studies that used prayer as a treatment in practice settings. He found that prayer had a positive effect in the outcome of illness, although the effect of prayer was not marked. Because of the results, Hodge concluded, "We should not be treating clients suffering with depression, for example, only with prayer. To treat depression, standard treatments, such as cognitive therapy, should be used as the primary method of treatment," but that prayer can be added to enhance the treatment and recovery from depression.

Psalms 42:2–6 includes a Jewish prayer for depression:

As the hart panteth after the water brooks, so panteth my soul after Thee, O God. My soul thirsteth for God, for the living God: "When shall I come and appear before God?" My tears have been my food day and night, while they say unto me all the day: "Where is Thy God?"

These things I remember, and pour out my soul within me, how I passed on with the throng, and led them to the house of God, with the voice of joy and praise, a multitude keeping holyday.

Why art thou cast down, O my soul? and why moanest thou within me? Hope thou in God; for I shall yet praise Him for the salvation of His countenance.

An example of a Muslim prayer for depression is as follows:

Oh Allah!
I am your servant,
son of Your male servant,
and son of Your female servant;
my forehead is in Your Hand;
Your judgment is exact;
Your decision about me is just;

I ask You by every name of Yours which You have called Yourself,
or revealed in a Book of Yours,
or taught to any of Your servants,
or reserved within Your unrevealed Knowledge,
to make the Qur'an a spring to my heart,
a light in my chest,
that it removes my sadness,
and erase my anguish.

(Saabiq 1991, 128)

Humor and Laughter for Depression

After ten years in therapy, my psychologist told me something very touching. He said, "No hablo ingles."

(Dennis Wolfberg)

In Proverbs 17:22, we read that "A merry heart doeth good like a medicine," and the Reader's Digest magazine proclaims, "Laughter is the best medicine." Modern research is showing why this is so. It appears that smiling and laughing lead to a reduction in cortisol, the stress chemical that is elevated in people with depression and increases the level of beta-endorphins (a naturally occurring brain chemical), which among other things is mood elevating.

Lee S. Berk, D.P.H., of Loma Linda University, has found that simply the anticipation of "mirthful laughter" involved in watching one's favorite funny movie leads to 27 percent more beta-endorphins and 87 percent more human growth hormone when compared with blood from the control group, which didn't anticipate the watching of a humorous video (Berk 2006). Like beta-endorphins, human growth hormone leads to a sense of well-being. There is some evidence that people with a better sense of humor live longer and healthier lives. The most obvious role of humor is its context in a person's social life: jokes, puns, and laughter often allow people to connect and to bond, to get along with the coworkers, friends, and others. Connection is vital from the point of view of mental health, because it reduces loneliness and, with it, depression. Research has shown that laughter boosts the immune system, which in turn increases natural disease-fighting killer cells and lowers blood pressure.

The Association for Applied and Therapeutic Humor (AATH) is an international community of nearly 600 therapists and other professionals who are interested in evidence-based research and practical applications of humor. They have defined what they call "therapeutic humor" as "any intervention that promotes health and wellness by stimulating a playful discovery, expression or appreciation of the absurdity or incongruity of life's situations" (www.aath.org).

Laughter appears to work to improve mood, but research shows that even "forced laughter" can have mood-elevating effects. Charles Schaefer, Ph.D., professor of psychology at Fairleigh Dickinson University, and colleagues (Schaefer 2002) have found that forced laughter is a powerful, readily available, cost-free tool for people to boost their mood and psychological well-being. In the research, Schaefer first asked his research subjects questions that measured their mood. He then directed them to laugh heartily for a minute and tested them again. On average, test subjects reported feeling significantly better after sixty seconds of forced laughter. The theory is that, once the brain signals the body to laugh, the body doesn't care why it is laughing. It's going to release endorphins, which is going to relieve stress as a natural physiological response to the physical act of laughing.

Before moving on to the "mechanical therapies," it seems fitting to end with a joke told me by a supervisor while I was in training:

A man receiving psychotherapy for depression goes to see his psychiatrist, and says: "Doctor, I'm feeling depressed and feeling somewhat suicidal. What should I do?"

The psychiatrist replies, "Pay your bill today."

MECHANICAL AND ELECTRICAL CURES

In the early 1900s, Europe was plagued with syphilis, a bacteria that causes a sexually transmitted disease that leads to terrible rashes, ulcers, warts, bowel, bladder, kidney, liver, and joint problems. Ultimately, it infects the whole body if untreated and can kill the infected person. If the infection reaches the brain, it can lead to the person developing personality changes, violence, and depression.

In 1917, Austrian psychiatrist Julius Wagner von Jauregg injected patients who had a syphilitic infection of the brain with malaria. The malaria caused a very high fever and convulsions in these patients. The high fever killed the syphilis bacteria and the patients improved. This led to the treatment and cure of thousands of syphilis-infected patients locked up in the lunatic asylums of the time. For this discovery, he won the Nobel Prize for medicine.

Nearly a decade later, Manfred Joshua Sakel, a Polish psychiatrist, discovered the "insulin coma therapy" for schizophrenics and other mental patients. He noted that giving these patients insulin would dramatically drop their blood sugar, which would in turn cause them to have a seizure. When the patients came out of the seizure, their mood had improved markedly. The procedure was so successful that, soon after he described his findings, insulin coma therapy became commonplace.

This leads us to the story of another Nobel Laureate, that of John Nash, the mathematician who won the Nobel Prize for economics and whose life story was made famous in the movie *A Beautiful Mind*. Nash first showed clear signs of schizophrenia in 1959 while teaching at the Massachusetts Institute of Technology. He was involuntarily committed to the McLean Hospital near Boston. After his stay there, he tried to return to work when fellow academics arranged a teaching appointment at Princeton University. Sadly, his illness worsened, and he was rehospitalized, this time at Trenton State Hospital in New Jersey. He underwent six weeks of insulin coma treatment, which led to a marked improvement, and he was able to once again return to work. Unfortunately, one major problem with insulin coma therapy was that, although people rapidly improved, the improvement did not last long, and the symptoms of mental illness rapidly returned.

It was because of this that research continued into finding safer and more long-lasting therapies for depression and other mental disorders. In 1934, Ladislas Joseph von Meduna, a Hungarian psychiatrist, gave intravenous injections of metrazol, a drug that causes severe and violent seizures, to schizophrenics and depressed patients. Once again, a large majority of the patients improved. Once again, the procedure became a widespread treatment. Once again, however, the effects of the metrazol were so horrific that, despite patients improving, few wanted to experience the treatment.

It was clear that convulsions appeared to be clearing up the fog, confusion, and depression of the mentally ill but that the ways in which the seizures had been induced led to intolerable side effects or only short-term improvement. In 1938, Dr. Ugo Cerletti, an Italian neurologist, witnessed that pigs about to be butchered were prepared for slaughter by being electrically shocked through the temples prior to meeting their fate. This rendered the pigs unconscious but did not kill them. He decided to try this on his psychiatric patients, and he found that the electric shocks caused his obsessive and difficult mental patients to become calm and manageable.

In all of these treatments, a seizure was used to improve the mental functioning and lives of psychiatric patients. Of all four methods, the "shock therapy" was considered the safest and became the most widely used. Electroconvulsive therapy (ECT) came of age.

ECT

In her book *Shock: The Healing Power of Electroconvulsive Therapy*, Kitty Dukakis (the wife of former presidential nominee Michael Dukakis), divulged not only that she had suffered from depression but also that she had received ECT to treat the depression. She wrote the following:

> It is not an exaggeration to say that electroconvulsive therapy has opened a new reality for me. As important, ECT has gotten me off anti-depressants. I withdrew slowly, with help from my doctors. Since I have been off I know the full range of my feelings. I get into the car now and put on music, the classical station. I sometimes cry because it conjures up feelings of my dad, who died on March 29, 2003, and was a conductor of the Boston Pops. Once I went off antidepressants, I finally could grieve.
>
> (Dukakis and Tye 2006)

ECT is a procedure frequently used to treat severe depression when other treatments such as medications have failed. In patients with delusions such as paranoia, hallucinations such as hearing voices, or persistent suicidal thoughts, ECT can be life saving.

TV host Dick Cavett once said about ECT, "In my case, ECT was miraculous. My wife was dubious, but when she came into my room afterward, I sat up and said, 'Look who's back among the living.' It was like a magic wand."

Changes to the ECT procedure over decades of use have made it a very safe treatment, although its past reputation including its use as a "cure" for homosexuality has given ECT its share of controversy. At the end of 1951, the CIA was very interested in learning techniques for brainwashing. They recognized that electroshock treatments could produce amnesia for varying lengths of time and that information could be obtained from patients as they came out of the stupor that followed shock treatments. Furthermore, depending on the electrical setting, the electroshock machine cold provide a shock that led to excruciating pain that, although not therapeutic, could be effective to get someone to talk. In Canada, psychiatrist Donald Cameron used the Page-Russell technique of powerful and intensive shocks to so-called "depattern" his patients. In particular, the idea was that "after the war each surviving German over the age of twelve should receive a short course of electroshock treatment to burn out any remaining vestige of Nazism." It later emerged that the CIA had in part funded his experiments.

Other than the controversy, another potential problem for ECT was its use as depicted in movies. The most famous portrayal of ECT on film was in *One Flew Over the Cuckoo's Nest*. In the movie, there is an attempt to get the patient McMurphy (played by Jack Nicholson) to comply with the rules by giving him ECT without an anesthetic. "This won't hurt a bit and it will be over in just a minute," he is told. After a pincer set of electrodes is placed on his temples, a switch is flicked on the ECT machine and McMurphy immediately begins a very disturbing, violent and painful seizure. ECT is presented as a barbaric and unjustified tool for social control and is also depicted as impotent and ineffective.

Modern-day ECT patients are given anesthesia and muscle relaxants. After the patient is relaxed, an electrical current is applied to the scalp through electrodes placed on the temples or elsewhere on the head. This electrical stimulation, which lasts up to eight seconds, produces a short seizure in the patient. One significant side effect of contemporary ECT is short-term memory loss. Ernest Hemingway, who committed suicide shortly after receiving ECT treatment at the famed Mayo Clinic in Minnesota, once said, "Well, what is the sense of ruining my head and erasing my memory, which is my capital, and putting me out of business?"

This problem can be lessened by unilateral ECT, which is an electrical current applied to one side of the head rather than bilateral ECT, which is when the electrical current is applied to both sides of the head. In general, ECT treatments are done two to three times a week for two to three weeks and are usually given in combination with medication and psychotherapy. This combination can work wonders.

Vagal Nerve Stimulation

In 1744, the French Royal Academic Society published a report entitled *Electricity and Medicine* and continued to publish it every second year thereafter. A 1755 account described how the application of electricity to a patient resulted in a convulsion in the patient, which in turn led to the cure of his hysterical blindness, which is a rare psychological condition in which severe stress results in a person believing that they cannot see. The idea of somehow applying electricity to the brain to cure it of its ails has been compelling for a long time, but electricity was always delivered from outside the body. Was it possible to get inside the body and use actual nerves to carry the electrical activity to the brain?

Cranial nerves are nerves that emerge directly from the brain. These nerves are different from spinal nerves, which emerge from the spinal cord. There are a total of twelve cranial nerves. The vagus nerve is the tenth cranial nerve. It starts in the brainstem and travels down below the neck to the abdomen. It is responsible for such varied tasks as controlling heart rate, controlling the contractions of the intestines and the stomach, sweating, and some of the muscle movements in the mouth, including speech.

VNS was initially developed for the treatment of a specific type of epilepsy. The idea behind VNS is that a small electrical shock is delivered to the vagus nerve by a stopwatch-sized generator that is implanted just under the skin in the left chest area. It then delivers preprogrammed, mild, intermittent electrical pulses to the vagus nerve twenty-four hours a day, and this was shown to reduce some types of seizures. Some patients, however, also reported an improvement in mood with the VNS system, and so it was investigated for depression.

By applying a small shock to the nerve in the chest, the shock is relayed as a nerve impulse to the limbic system, which in large part deals with mood, motivation, sleep, appetite, and alertness. In 2005, the FDA approved the device in patients older than eighteen with treatment-resistant depression or those who had been treated with, but failed to respond to, four adequate antidepressant trials and/or ECT treatment. However, not all patients responded to the VNS, and some actually got worse. Because of this, it is neither widely recommended by psychiatrists, nor requested by patients.

Transcranial Magnetic Stimulation

Franz Anton Mesmer was an eighteenth-century German mathematician and physician, who wrote his doctoral thesis on the effects of gravitational fields on human health. Even long before Mesmer, Cleopatra was reported to have worn a naturally magnetic lodestone on her forehead to slow down the aging process. Mesmer suggested that there was magnetic energy flowing throughout the universe as well as inside the body and that it was the flow of this magnetic energy, when disrupted, that caused mental illnesses like depression. He experimented with using magnets to treat seizures and mental illnesses. He was a theatrical charmer who traveled around Europe and opened a magnetism salon in Paris. There, patients sat in water-filled vats containing iron filings and rods and would pour magnetic water on parts of their bodies affected by illness to facilitate the magnetic flow. They sometimes fainted or went into convulsions and later claimed that they were "mesmerized" by Mesmer (from whom the word is derived).

Perhaps the Mesmer of nearly 300 years ago was onto something when he considered the therapeutic benefits of magnets. The word magnet comes from the ancient Greeks. It is derived from Magnes lithos, or the "stone from Magnesia," an area of Greece that was known for its volcanic rocks with magnetic properties. Today's magnetic health applications involve neither volcanoes nor spas. Transcranial magnetic stimulation (TMS) is an experimental procedure that uses magnetic fields to alter brain activity. The FDA has not approved TMS. Although it is unclear how it works, it has been shown that magnetic fields alter brain function. Generally, in trials, a large electromagnetic coil is held against the skull near the forehead. An electric current creates a magnetic pulse that travels through the skull and into the brain. The magnetic pulse causes small electrical currents, which in turn stimulate nerve cells in the parts of the brain involved in mood regulation and depression. The procedure is different from VNS in that no surgery or device implantation is involved, and the outpatient treatment would be carried out over three to six weeks in weekly thirty-minute sessions.

Although the FDA has not approved this treatment, some patients swear by the health benefits of magnets, and one patient told me that their depression had been completely cured by sleeping on a mattress embedded with magnets. It is hard to imagine that we won't continue to investigate the potential benefits of such an intriguing therapy.

Deep Brain Stimulation

If ECT was developed to apply electricity from outside the head to influence the brain and the VNS to apply electricity from a nerve inside the body to the brain, perhaps it is not surprising that the next move would be to move inside the brain itself. Here is how it works. First, there is an operation in which two holes are drilled into the skull and the surgeon implants electrodes in the brain. (The idea of drilling holes into the skull has come full circle since the ancient practice of trepanation!) In a second operation, a neurostimulator device is implanted into the chest. Finally, wires from the brain electrodes are placed under the skin and guided down to the neurostimulator in the chest. The neurostimulator then sends electrical pulses along the wires to the electrodes in the brain, stimulating those areas.

The theory behind this treatment is that an electrical current can directly stimulate certain parts of the brain in an attempt to change mood. Deep brain stimulation is regularly used in people with Parkinson's disease. Despite this, the FDA has not approved the procedure for use in depression. In part, this is because one of the major side effects of the procedure is, in fact, depression.

Light Therapy

Hippocrates would be pleasantly surprised at how, after 2,000 years, just how many of his observations and interventions are still referenced today or still practiced today. With regard to the use of light, probably the most remarkable insight was the positive influence of sunlight on mental health. Hippocrates recognized that depression was more common in the winter months in Greece when there was less sunlight. In 200 AD, Ptolemy observed that patterns of color rays coming from the sun into the eyes produced a feeling of euphoria. In 1806, psychiatrist Philippe Pinel identified two types of seasonal depression, one occurring in winter and another in summer. By 1845, his student Jean-Etienne Esquirol, who would later be recognized as the "father of French psychiatry," documented several cases of both types of depression. In the late nineteenth and early twentieth centuries, bright light was frequently prescribed for a number of mood- and stress-related disorders. Prior to World War II, hospitals were regularly built with solariums, or sun rooms, in which patients could spend time recuperating in the sunlight. After that, the so-called "light bath" became popular in Europe; "heliotherapy" it was called, after Helios, the Greek god of the sun. During the twentieth century, light therapy would be rediscovered several times as an effective means for treating SADs.

Today, light therapy is a standard treatment for SAD. Mary, a thirty-three-year-old mother of three spent winters feeling "down in the dumps" until her depressive illness was diagnosed as SAD. The dread of facing winter brought her to the point of suicidality. She said, "I was so depressed. I could not understand what was happening to my mind, and the thought of winter coming made me even more terrified. I was constantly exhausted, and at one point I was admitted to a psychiatric hospital." Despite being treated for clinical depression with antidepressants, it was not until she had started light therapy that her symptoms improved. Despite many studies showing the effectiveness of light therapy, the FDA has not given approval to market light boxes for the treatment of SAD.

Research has shown that SAD probably arises from abnormalities in the levels of the brain chemical melatonin. Melatonin helps to control body temperature, the secretion of other hormones, and sleep. During the low-light months of fall and winter, people with SAD produce more melatonin than normal, which can at times lead to severe depression. Exposure to bright light, such as that from a light box, has been shown in some studies to reduce the production of melatonin, thereby reducing the symptoms of SAD. With new light boxes, people suffering from SAD require two weeks of sitting under the light for thirty minutes to get a therapeutic response.

When light, electricity, chemistry, and talk fail to relieve a depression that becomes progressively more severe, it can be time to consider going under the knife.

BRAIN SURGERY TO TREAT DEPRESSION

Much of the controversy surrounding the use of brain surgery to treat depression and other psychiatric conditions is attributed to a history of indiscriminate use and the high incidence of side effects seen with the early procedures. Perhaps the experience of Rosemary Kennedy would have been enough to dissuade others from the consideration of brain surgery to treat depression, but research into surgical approaches continued. Brain surgery continued to be considered because, although it became increasingly clear that the therapeutic approach to depression involved a combination of psychotherapy, medication, and at times ECT, many patients failed to respond adequately and remained severely disabled.

Today, only patients with severe, chronic and disabling depression and those who have not responded to repeated standard treatment or alternative options are considered for surgical intervention and only after the risks and benefits of the brain surgery have been clearly reviewed by the patient and the patient's loved ones. Only once it is determined that the person's depression remains debilitating and that their life-functioning could be improved, and if no other therapy is viable is surgery then offered. A variety of brain operations are considered for depression.

Stereotactic Subcaudate Tractotomy

In 1991, Kartsounis and colleagues at Guy's Hospital in London reported a study on the ominous sounding "stereotactic subcaudate tractotomy," a surgical procedure performed for the treatment of unrelenting depression and other mood disorders. The surgery involves the destruction of the nerve pathways between the frontal lobes and the head of the caudate nucleus. The caudate nucleus is an important part of the brain's learning and memory system. In their study, they reported the results of the operation in twenty-three patients (sixteen of whom had depression) and found that the operation did not cause any significant, long-term adverse, cognitive deficits. In a review of all the studies in which this procedure has been used to treat depression, the response rate is 55–68 percent of patients getting better. The patients did however have a tendency to "confabulate," which is a tendency to fill in gaps in a person's memory with fabrications that the person believes to be facts. Furthermore, the swelling that occurred in the frontal lobes after the operation led to a decrease in executive functioning. Depression has been the most common diagnosis for patients undergoing this technique.

Limbic Leucotomy

Neurosurgeon Desmond Kelly introduced the procedure known as "limbic leucotomy" in 1973. It combined the aforementioned subcaudate tractotomy with a procedure known as anterior cingulotomy, which had been shown to be effective for treating unbearable pain that does not respond to standard treatments. Kelly reasoned that these two operations might lead to a better result for the symptoms of depression than either operation alone.

Research shows that, in depression 50–78 percent of patients improve. Interestingly although patients complain of lethargy, confusion, and lack of sphincter control in the early postoperative period, ongoing or serious complications are rare. Twelve percent of patients do complain of persistent lethargy. Another interesting finding is that patient IQ showed slight improvement after the operation.

Anterior Capsulotomy

The French neurosurgeon Jean Talairach described the operation known as an anterior capsulotomy in 1949. The Swedish neurosurgeon Lars Leksell popularized the procedure for patients with a variety of psychiatric disorders. The aim of the operation was to cut the connections between the frontal lobes and the thalamus. Research shows that this operation leads to increased activity and improved attention in patients. In the first 116 patients operated on by Leksell, forty-eight percent of depressed patients had a satisfactory response.

Complications of the surgery include confusion during the first week as well as nighttime bladder control problems. Some patients experience a recurrence of depression, and, in one case, a patient committed suicide after the operation. Other patients experience excessive fatigue. Finally, weight gain is common after capsulotomy, with an overall mean weight gain of about 10 percent in all patients.

A New Kind of Knife

Recognizing that using a surgeon's scalpel to cut into the brain had a risk of significant complications, Leksell developed what he would call a "gamma knife." Gamma knife surgery is unique in that no surgical incision is made to expose the inside of the brain. This significantly reduces the risk of surgical complications and eliminates the side effects and dangers of general anesthesia. The "blades" of the gamma knife are beams of gamma radiation programmed to target a specific point in the brain. In a single treatment session, exactly 201 beams of gamma radiation focus precisely on the target point. Individually, none of these 201 beams hurt the brain as they pass through its tissue, but the combined effect of all 201 beams leads to the destruction of the specific target. Thus, the gamma knife "cuts" deep into the brain without using a scalpel.

In one report, an outpatient gamma knife operation was performed for treatment of intractable depression. The patient had undergone over 300 electroshock therapies and 52 different inpatient medication trials without relief of her depression. She was referred for a gamma knife subcaudate tractotomy, which led to a complete resolution of her depression.

Although historically any patient with a severe psychiatric illness was considered a candidate for surgical intervention, today the indications for psychosurgery are more restrictive. Under these conditions, many patients improve markedly after surgery, and the complications or side effects are few. Brain surgery has therefore become an important therapeutic option for disabling psychiatric disease.

Often times, however, because of lack of access, lack of information, lack of resources, or a desire for a completely different approach, patients turn away from the aforementioned approaches and move to an "alternative" solution.

ALTERNATIVE APPROACHES TO TREATING DEPRESSION

Herbs and Vitamins

Gladys was a forty-two-year-old saleswoman from Boston who had been active until a year ago when she shattered her right leg in a skiing accident. She had been told to expect to be in a cast for sixteen weeks, but she developed an infection and her recovery time was a lot longer than anticipated. Eventually the fracture healed, but she noticed that she lost much of her energy or desire to be with people. The thought of going for her annual hike in the White Mountains with her friends no longer appealed. Her sales started to drop off at work, and her boss noted that she wasn't her "chipper, usual self." Her personality had guaranteed success in a job that required a "sunny disposition," but she became increasingly gloomy and found it hard to smile or to get excited about the prospect of a sale.

At home, her husband and teenage daughters were worried but uncertain about what to do other than encouraging her to "do the things she wanted to do," but Gladys recognized that she didn't particularly want to do anything. She had always been a health-conscious person and carefully watched what she ate, did not eat red meat, and always chose "natural" foods. Despite being thin, she had started to lose her appetite and lost some weight.

At the bidding of her family doctor, she finally agreed to see a psychiatrist who diagnosed her with depression and prescribed a course of antidepressants. She refused to take these because she did not "believe" in a chemical solution but told the psychiatrist that she would consider a "natural remedy." The doctor told Gladys that the FDA had not approved any "natural" or "alternative" medications for the treatment of depression. Her psychiatrist did, however, mention that there was some research being done on the so-called alternative treatments. Gladys spent some time researching these and then went to a health food store, where she was told about omega-3 fatty acids. After doing her own "research," Gladys started taking the recommended dose every morning and, after four weeks, felt that her mood was lifting, that she was feeling calmer, that her sleep, appetite, and energy had improved, and that she even looked forward to going to work. Given her overall improvement, she continued to take the omega-3 supplements and went on a belated hike with her friends.

Many people who suffer from depression choose not to take antidepressant medication. Some cannot tolerate the side effects, others are worried that the medications will cause suicidal thinking, and yet others say that they will only take "natural" remedies. These natural remedies come in the form of fish oils, amino acids or proteins, and plant extracts or herbs.

For as many years as the likes of Prozac and lithium have been around, nothing can top St. John's Wort (*Hypericum perforatum*) for longevity. It has been used for more than 2000 years to treat mental and other conditions!

The ancient Greeks and Romans used St. John's Wort to ward against evil spirits by placing sprigs of the plant on statues of their gods. The name *Hypericum* is from Greek meaning "over an apparition" because the herb was once considered smelly enough to cause evil spirits to depart. During medieval times, the Europeans used the plant to treat all forms of madness. It was sometimes referred to as herba demonis fuga, an herb to chase away the devil.

In 1618, the Pharmacopoeia Londinensis, a drug formulary of the time, listed an oil, made from the flowers of St. John's Wort, that was used to treat illnesses of the: "imagination, melancholia, anxiety and disturbances of understanding." Although St. John's Wort is the best known of the "herbal" treatments for depression, herbalists and nontraditional healers have recommended many other medication alternatives. The following is a list of the most commonly used to treat depression.

St. John's Wort

Most of the herbs marketed for depression have not undergone any serious scientific research. Of those with some support for its claim to treat depression, St. John's Wort appears to have credibility. Studies show that pharmaceutical-grade St. John's Wort extract effectively relieves depression and, in some studies, does as well in treating depression as approved antidepressants. However, because the FDA does not regulate St. John's Wort, the quality, purity, and dosage claims by the manufacturers of over-the-counter product is at times questionable. This is true of all of the drugs in this section.

Omega-3 Fatty Acids

Omega-3 fatty acids are essential to the growth and maintenance of brain cells, especially cell membranes. The human body cannot make omega-3 fatty acids and so these must be obtained from dietary sources. The most common dietary sources are fish, flax, and eggs from free-range chickens. Walnuts are another source of omega-3 fatty acids. Research has shown that there are very low omega-3 levels in the blood, cell membranes, and brains of depressed patients.

In 1996, the *Journal of the American Medical Association* published a study comparing the level of depression in the populations of ten nations. The results of the survey showed that depression varied tremendously by country. For instance, in Taiwan, 1.5 in every 100 adults experience depression compared with nineteen for every 100 adults in Lebanon. This study was followed by a studypublished in *The Lancet* that looked at how much fish was consumed in each of these ten nations (Hibbeln 1998). They found that the higher fish-consuming populations experienced less depression. Another study found that depression is sixty times higher in New Zealand, where the average consumption of seafood is forty pounds a year compared with Japan, where average per person consumption is nearly 150 pounds of seafood a year!

Harvard psychiatrist and researcher Dr. Andrew Stoll, author of *The Omega-3 Connection: The Groundbreaking Anti-Depression Diet and Brain Program*, has found that 1–3 grams of omega-3 per day had a remarkable effect in reducing depression (Stoll 2001). He has also warned against eating too much cold-ocean fish given that pollution has led to the accumulation of toxic levels of heavy metals in these fish.

Dehydroepiandrosterone

Interest in dehydroepiandrosterone (DHEA) rose after former home-run record holder Mark McGwire said he used androstenedione, or "andro," a similar supplement. DHEA is a naturally occurring steroid hormone that is a building block to the male sex hormone testosterone and the female sex hormone estrogen. It is made by the adrenal glands, but, starting in early adulthood, DHEA production starts to diminish. At age seventy, DHEA production is about 20 percent of that in the late teens or early twenties. Some studies have shown that it may be an effective treatment for major depression particularly in older adults. The hormone appears to work by increasing serotonin levels in the brain and blocking the effects of certain stress hormones, such as cortisol. Many researchers have felt that the risks of taking DHEA outweigh its "unproven" efficacy in depression. In particular, side effects such as oily skin, acne, deepening of the voice, overactivation, disinhibition, aggression, mania, or psychosis are concerning. In men, there is even further worry that DHEA increases prostate cancer.

Albizzia

To the Chinese, the Persian silk tree is known as "the tree of collective happiness." Its bark, *Cortex Albizzia julibrissin*, was written about in ancient herbal texts that described its ability to "promote joy, assuage sorrow, brighten the eye, and enliven the heart." It was prescribed (and continues to be prescribed) for anyone suffering from sadness or grief as a result of severe disappointment or loss and for emotional turmoil particularly when bad temper, depression, insomnia, and irritability was present. Research has shown that the flower of the silk tree also has a sedative effect. Because of these findings, some contemporary American Chinese herbalists have called it "herbal Prozac."

5-Hydroxytryptophan

5-Hydroxytryptophan (5-HTP) is the protein that is converted directly into serotonin, which as we have seen is considered to be deficient in clinical depression. Before we cover 5-HTP any further, there is a dark chapter in the history of nutritional supplements in the United States that indirectly relates to 5-HTP.

To understand what happened, a little biochemistry is essential. Amino acids are the building blocks of proteins. Essential amino acids are those amino acids that are essential to life but cannot be produced by humans. L-Tryptophan is an essential amino acid. Because we cannot produce it, it must come from our diet. L-Tryptophan is typically found in dietary proteins and is the chemical that is converted directly to 5-HTP, which as mentioned is then in turn converted to serotonin.

In the 1970s and 1980s, L-tryptophan was considered a staple in health food stores in the United States. It was heralded as a safe, non-addictive treatment for insomnia, premenstrual syndrome (PMS), and depression. Six Japanese manufacturers produced L-tryptophan for the U.S. market. One of the six producers, the petrochemical giant Showa Denko, controlled more than half of the American market. It sought to capture more of the market by boosting production, and they genetically engineered a bacterium called Strain V to produce huge quantities of L-tryptophan. Soon after this, the Centers for Disease Control (CDC) became aware of an outbreak of an extremely rare condition known as Eosinophilia-myalgia syndrome (EMS), which is a disorder that causes inflammation by white blood cells known as eosinophils in nerve, muscle, and connective tissue and can lead to swelling of the arms and legs, and the face. It can also cause joint pain, skin rashes, hair loss, cough, shortness of breath, and fatigue, and, in extreme conditions, this swelling can lead to death.

After several months of investigation, the EMS outbreak was traced back to the tryptophan made by Showa Denko. Their genetic tinkering apparently produced a toxic chemical. Tests showed that Showa Denko's L-tryptophan was 99.6 percent pure, but the tiny proportion of the compound that was considered "impure" contained between thirty and forty different contaminants, including a compound known as ethylidenebis L-tryptophan. This compound was shown to be the cause of EMS.

By 1990, the CDC confirmed over 1,500 cases of EMS, including thirty-eight deaths. This led the FDA to prohibit the importation of L-tryptophan and to issue a nationwide recall of all over-the-counter dietary supplements containing 100 milligrams or more of L-tryptophan. Since that time, L-tryptophan has made a comeback and, under more rigorous controls, is either manufactured in the United States or imported from what are considered to be reliable foreign suppliers.

This leads us back to 5-HTP. Given that it is the chemical that is formed just before becoming serotonin, researchers thought that it would be a safer option if a natural source could be found. It turns out to be plentiful in the *Griffonia simplicifolia* plant, a climbing shrub from central Africa. Today the plant is used widely as the major source of 5-HTP. Although research has shown that, taken in large quantities it can raise serotonin, taken at such high quantities can lead to nausea, vomiting, and severe diarrhea, which has limited its use, despite it having staunch adherents as a treatment for depression.

DL-Phenylalanine

Phenylalanine, like tryptophan, is an essential amino acid. In the body, phenylalanine is converted into a chemical known as L-tyrosine, which in turn is converted into L-dopa and then to dopamine, adrenaline, or noradrenaline. In Chapter 2, we saw how the levels of these last three chemicals (also known as neurotransmitters) are found to be low in people suffering from depression. Alternative health-food stores market DL-phenylalanine as a mood elevator, with the theory being that giving someone high doses of this building block of the aforementioned neurotransmitters will thereby increase their levels and thus relieve depression. Because there can be a buildup of adrenaline in people who take this supplement, common side effects are those of too much adrenaline and include elevated blood pressure, headache, irritability, aggressiveness, and difficulty falling asleep.

Tyrosine

Tyrosine is also an amino acid building block of adrenaline and noradrenaline. In one report (Goldberg 1980), two patients with long-standing depression who failed to respond to different medication trials as well as ECT were started on L-tyrosine and had their depression lift. In another case report, a thirty-year-old female with a two-year history of depression showed marked improvement after two weeks of treatment with L-tyrosine. Although these are interesting cases and the results were clearly beneficial to these individual patients, more robust research has failed to find any benefit to the use of tyrosine in depression.

Folate and Vitamin B12

Folate and vitamin B12 are required in the chemical reactions and the production of all the neurotransmitters. Both of these vitamins are plentiful and commonly found in fruits and leafy green vegetables. Deficiencies can, however, occur under certain circumstances, such as in the elderly and those with poor diets. Vitamin B12 deficiency is an issue for many older adults, with multiple factors such as poor diet, digestion problems, and drug interactions contributing to the problem.

People who have low blood levels of folate and vitamin B12 often present with psychiatric disturbances including depression. Some studies have shown that up to one-third of people with depression have low folate levels. Other research has shown that people who did not have enough folate responded less quickly to antidepressant medication than people with normal folate levels. Folic acid appears to accelerate the onset of the therapeutic effect of some antidepressants. Because of these findings and certainly in the elderly, the addition of a multivitamin with folate and B12 is often a reasonable consideration.

S-Adenosylmethionine

There is a chemical reaction known as methylation. In the human body, this chemical reaction is essential for maintaining active neurotransmitters, including serotonin, dopamine, and hormones. The process is essential for maintaining phospholipids (the fats that make up the walls of nerve cells in the brain). For methylation to occur, various chemicals are necessary, and of all of these, S-adenosylmethionine (SAMe) is the most important methylating agent in the brain.

Many studies have shown that, when used as a dietary supplement, SAMe may have beneficial effects on mood. Of all the so-called "natural" remedies, SAMe appears to have the most convincing scientific evidence as an antidepressant. It alleviates the symptoms of depression when used alone or to-gether with antidepressant medication. It also appears to work faster than the four to six weeks generally considered for a typical antidepressant. Side effects are rare, generally mild, and include gastric upset with nausea and vomiting, and, if used at high concentrations, it may also cause dry mouth, restlessness, and anxiety.

Vitamin B6

Vitamin B6 is found in a wide variety of foods, including fortified cereals, beans, meat, poultry, fish, and some fruits and vegetables. It is an essential part of more than 100 enzymes involved in protein metabolism. It is also essential for red blood cell metabolism. The nervous and immune systems need vitamin B6 to function efficiently.

Because of this, researchers have tested it in people with depression. Again, as with some of the other vitamins, there was no evidence that it alleviated depression. However, with more careful scrutiny of the research, it appears that B6 may have a role in alleviating the low mood state associated with the PMS. Not all studies have shown this benefit, and even those studies that have shown the benefit warn that taking an excess of B6 can result in nerve damage to the arms and legs. It is true, however, that taking too much of any-thing is generally not a good thing!

Alternative Nonherbal Therapies

Many people either do not want to take medication or cannot tolerate the side effects of medication. Their depression is not so severe that ECT or some other invasive procedure is needed, but yet their depression interferes with their enjoyment of life. Even the idea of taking herbal remedies smacks of altering brain chemistry unnaturally. Other than psychotherapy, patients have used the following alternative therapies to treat their depression. In Chapter 2, we considered cultural differences in the conceptualization of depression. Some of these alternative treatments are used almost exclusively by individual cultures, and other practices have become more widespread in their use.

Native American Traditional Practices

By 1890, in the United States, the Lakota and other Indians of the Great Plains had been militarily defeated and most were living impoverished lives on reservations. At that time, a Native American prophet known as Wovoka from the Paiute tribe of the Southwest foretold that a great storm in the form of a whirlwind would come in the spring of 1891, covering over the earth with new earth and burying the old, corrupt, and unjust world, and from there a beautiful new and just world would arise.

According to Wovoka, all the Indians had to do to create this paradise was to believe in it and to participate in a special ceremonial dance known as the Ghost Dance. This dance would make them as light as a feather, and, when the storm came, they would simply float above it until the earth had settled.

Although the Ghost Dance never produced its desired effect, for many Native Americans it was a way of recovering hope and battling against the despair and depression of having had their lives and lands taken away from them. To this day, ceremonial dances like the Ghost Dance as well as chants and cleansing rituals are part of Indian Health Service programs to heal depression, stress, trauma, and substance abuse.

Acupuncture

Acupuncture is an ancient Chinese procedure that has been used for more than 2000 years to treat specific illnesses or conditions. The therapist sticks very fine, solid metallic needles into specific points on the body. The theory is that this process stimulates the body's ability to heal illnesses and conditions by correcting imbalances. The body is seen in traditional Chinese medicine as a delicate balance of two opposing and inseparable forces, yin and yang, and that when these are not in balance illness occurs. From a more Western perspective, it is considered that acupuncture prompts the body to produce chemicals that decrease or eliminate painful sensations, including depression.

Reflexology

This is a technique in which a therapist applies pressure to specific points, most commonly on the feet, but also on the hands and ears, to encourage a beneficial effect on some other part of the body. Reflexologists believe that the body has the capacity to heal itself and that the foot is divided into a number of reflex zones corresponding to the zones of the energy in other parts of the body. It is believed that, by applying pressure in the form of a deep massage to the reflex zone that is tight, the healing process is stimulated and the body and mind ultimately heals itself.

Meditation

Meditation is a practice in which a person works with their mental state to effect the desired change. The basic concept is that, with awareness, we can, to a certain degree, choose how to respond to circumstances. Meditation practice calms the mind and helps develops positive emotions. It helps to develop an awareness of the impermanence and interconnectedness of our experience. If a person recognizes irritability and impatience in their mental state, they might work on relaxation through slow breathing and awareness of their mental state and let go of the hurtful emotions. It works best when practiced regularly for fifteen or more minutes a day. For some, while the body is at rest, the mind is cleared by focusing on a thought, a word, a phrase, or a scenery. Others practice meditation during some rituls in their life, such as brushing their teeth. Interestingly, although meditation is most closely associated with Buddhism, almost all the major religions have some sort of meditative practice.

Exercise

Gerry was a forty-six-year-old Seattle man who lapsed into what he described as a terrible funk over the past few weeks and was worried that he would slip into a full depression, a condition that had plagued his family for many generations. He tried medication but it stunted his libido, which made him more depressed, so he stopped taking the medication. Yet he knew he had to do something. He had also gained about twenty pounds since his days in college where he had run for the cross-country team. Although initially he found getting out of the house to be a chore, he ran for three miles five days a week and, after three weeks, recognized that his mood had improved and he had begun to lose weight.

Research has found that thirty minutes of aerobic workouts of moderate intensity, three to five times weekly, cut mild to moderate depression symptoms nearly in half. These research findings are comparable with other psychiatric treatments such as medication and psychotherapy.

The theory is that exercise increases the levels of mood-enhancing neurotransmitters in the brain and boosts endorphins, a natural opiate-like substance, that makes people feel good. Other research has shown that running leads to new nerve formation in the hippocampus and that this nerve growth is beneficial as an antidepressant in a genetic animal model of depression and in depressed humans. Exercise also appears to work by reducing muscle tension, improving sleep quality, and reducing levels of the stress hormone cortisol. It also increases body temperature, which may have calming effects. The cumulative effect of these changes can be a reduction in sadness, anxiety, irritability, stress, fatigue, and anger.

Guided Imagery and Relaxation

Guided imagery is a form of focused relaxation that can enhance a person's coping skills. It coaches a person to mentally create a calm, peaceful image that can be called upon for therapeutic purposes, a mental place where a person cannot be hurt. People generally choose a place such as a lake, a beach, or a mountain or an enjoyable event such as time spent with friends or family. Research has shown that such imagery works best when used together with a relaxation technique. Yoga is the most common relaxation technique used with imagery.

Imagery had been found to be very effective for the treatment of stress, and the practice of imagery is thought to release neurotransmitters, which, as in exercise, leads to the lowering of blood pressure, heart rate, and anxiety levels.

Massage

Massage uses touch through gentle pressure, kneading tight muscles and stroking the skin to provide relaxation. For pregnant women who are reluctant to take antidepressant medications during their pregnancy and who have limited access to psychotherapy, massage therapy appears to have some benefit. Research has shown that depressed adolescent mothers who received ten thirty-minute massage sessions have an overall reduction in anxiety levels and a reduction in stress hormones. As in the other techniques, the goal of relaxation appears to be central to obtaining anxiety and stress reduction, which can aggravate depression.

Prayer and Faith

A colleague shared with me the case of Camille, a deeply religious twenty-seven-year-old woman who was suffering with clinical depression. She had been in contact with him by e-mail due to the great distance from his practice in Anchorage, Alaska.

She wrote, "I am suffering from a deep depression but I am trying to keep positive. We [the family] have prayer every evening here at home, but I do feel useless and worthless. Although I know that my depression is biological I think that only God can totally cure me. I am waiting for the package of meds that you sent me to arrive, but perhaps you could also pray for me."

Although in a secular society it is often taboo to talk about prayer, it is also true that people often turn to their faith for help during times of need and ill health, including depression. There is, however, some research that prayer may help to overcome depression.

Research shows, for instance, that moderate levels of prayer and other types of religious coping may help combat depression among spouses of people with lung cancer (Abernathy et al. 2002). The study included 156 spouses of people with various stages of lung cancer. The spouses were twenty-six to eighty-five years old, and 78 percent of them were women. The researchers assessed the spouses' levels of religious belief and religious practices, such as prayer, as well as their level of depression, along with their sense of control over events and level of social support. They found that spouses who used moderate levels of religious coping were less depressed than spouses who used lower or higher levels of religious coping.

It might seem counterintuitive that a high level of religious coping is associated with more depression. One thought in this connection is that an over-reliance on religion leads to neglect of other important coping strategies.

In another study (Koenig, George, and Peterson 1998), the researchers looked at the effects of religious belief and religious activity on remission of depression in medically ill hospitalized older patients. They interviewed patients aged sixty years or over who had been admitted to medical inpatient services and assessed their level of depression. A total of ninety-four were found to have a depressive disorder. After hospital discharge, depressed patients were followed up by telephone at twelve-week intervals four times. At each follow-up contact, the patients were asked about their depression and about their religious practices. At the end of the study, 54 percent of the patients no longer had symptoms of depression. Interestingly, the more faith a person had, the quicker the time to recovery, but simply attending church did little to increase the time to remission of depression.

Cuentos (Stories) for Children

Based on folktales, this form of therapy originated in Puerto Rico. The stories are told by the therapists and contain healing themes and models of behavior such as self-transformation and endurance through adversity. *Cuentos* are often used to help Latino children recover from depression and other mental health problems, especially those related to leaving their homeland and living in a foreign culture.

All of these treatment methods, whether traditional, nontraditional, or a combination of both, have a common goal and that is to treat depression. Leaving depression untreated can have some very serious consequences that extend beyond its effect on the individual alone.

5

Complications of Depression

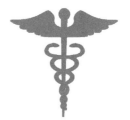

Suicide is a permanent solution to a temporary problem.

(Gold 1986, 290)

SUICIDE

Nearly 30,000 Americans commit suicide every year; 650,000 receive emergency treatment after a suicide attempt. A further tragedy is that about 90 percent of those suicides are due to treatable disorders, the most common of which is depression. Statistics show that people with depression have up to a 15 percent risk for suicide. A report on suicide by the U.S. surgeon general (1999) states that, "major depressive disorders account for about 20–35 percent of all deaths by suicide" and moreover that depressed men are more likely to commit suicide than depressed women.

The majority of people who suffer from depression do not commit suicide. They choose instead to struggle with the suffering while looking for answers. For many, however, the thought of suicide sadly persists as the only solution to the problem. In 2005, twenty-one-year-old Australian golfer Steven Bowditch won the Jacob's Creek Open in Adelaide. It was a huge win for the

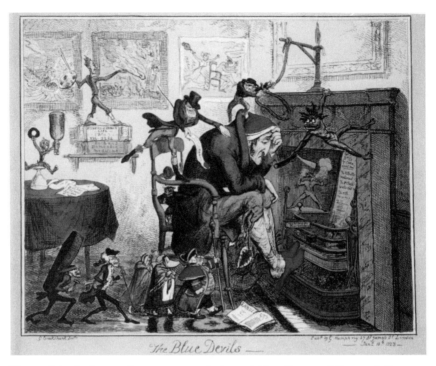

Figure 5.1. A depressed man contemplating suicide. *Courtesy Library of Congress, Prints & Photographs Division, LC-USZC2-614.*

young golfer who looked to follow fellow Australian golfing great Greg Norman to the United States to make his fortune on the lucrative American golf circuit. Tragically, he succumbed to a crippling depression, which nearly destroyed more than just his golfing and life dreams. After starting a course of antidepressant medication, he gave a newspaper interview to the *Herald Sun* in 2006 in which he said the following:

> Golf at this stage of my life is not a concern to me. It's my well being off the course. The biggest problem is off the golf course. That's when it really hurts. I went a stretch of 13 days where I didn't have a wink of sleep. You get thoughts you shouldn't have, your being on tour, your purpose of living over here, living in general. They are questions you ask yourself I don't wish on anyone.

His thoughts echo those of Mike Wallace, the CBS TV host of 60 *Minutes*, when Wallace said this "At first I couldn't sleep, then I couldn't eat. I felt hopeless and I just couldn't cope ... and then I just lost all perspective on things. You know, you become crazy. I had done a story for *60 Minutes* on depression previously, but I had no idea that I was now experiencing it. Finally, I collapsed and just went to bed." In the interview, he revealed that he had attempted suicide with an overdose of pills.

Fame and Wealth Are No Protection

What do the books *The Old Man and the Sea*, *The Bell Jar*, the painting *Starry Nights*, the poem "Love Songs," and the song "Smells Like Teen Spirit" all have in common? Their composers Ernest Hemingway, Sylvia Plath, Vincent van Gogh, Sara Teasdale, and Kurt Cobain all suffered from depression and committed suicide. So too have millions of equally well known, lesser known, and completely unknown sufferers of depression. In his book *Suicide: The Forever Decision*, psychologist Paul G. Quinnett, Ph.D., writes, "Research has shown that a substantial majority of people have considered suicide at one time in their lives, and I mean considered it seriously" (Quinnett 1993, 12).

The list of well known people who have suffered from depression and committed suicide is so extensive that the names alone would fill this book and many others. Here are some other more or less familiar names: the writers Charlotte Perkins Gilman and James Robert Baker; the composers Peter Warlock, Oskar Nedbal, and Peter Tchaikovsky; the musicians Vince Welnick and Gary Stewart; the poets Thomas Chatterton, John Gould Fletcher, and Anne Sexton; the artists, Iris von Roten-Meyer, Mark Lombardi, and Robert Bishop; the actors Margaux Hemingway, Elizabeth Hartman, Jonathan Brandis, and Marilyn Monroe; the senators Robert La Follette and Jesse Thomas; the athletes Luis Ocana, Marc Potvin, and Terry Long; the presidents Getulio Dornelles Vargas and Carlos Roberto Reina; the psychologists Bruno Bettelheim and Michel Gauquelin; and the doctors Jonathan Drummond-Webb and Harold Shipman.

Aristotle was most observant when he noted, "Why is it that all those who have become eminent in philosophy or politics, or poetry or the arts are clearly melancholics, and some of them to such an extent as to be affected by diseases caused by black bile?" (Forster 1984).

When depressed suicidal patients talk about the suicidal thinking, they often say that it is less about ending the misery of the depression than ending the loneliness they feel. "It's hard for me to put into words the horrific feeling of being depressed. It is the most sickening feeling in the world when you believe you are miserable and you're all alone," said Terry Bradshaw, NFL Hall of Fame quarterback (Morgan 2004).

For many patients, it is this loneliness that accompanies depression that kills, and so it is not surprising that many people have attributed the love and caring of those close to them for saving them from suicide. Tennis great Pat Cash, the 1987 Wimbledon champion, once told the press, "There are times I've been very close to committing suicide. Only the fact that I have children has stopped me. Looking back I can see that underlying depression was there, even during my teens." Children and the love of a family is one major reason suicidal patients offer as to why they won't kill themselves. Mark Twain too recognized this when he wrote in a letter to fellow author William Dean Howells, "I do see that there is an argument against suicide: the grief of the worshipers left behind, the awful famine in their hearts, these are too costly terms for the release."

Losing the Battle: The Notes Left Behind

Depression is cancer of the emotions.

(Wolpert 2000)

Some with severe depression, like some with a rapidly spreading cancer, lose the will and capacity to live. Different from cancer, which can be seen under a microscope in a laboratory, the only postmortem clue to depression is at times the note left behind by the suicidal person. It is commonly thought that most people who commit suicide leave notes, but only 15–25 percent of those who kill themselves leave suicide notes. The purpose of the notes falls into five broad categories:

1. To explain the reason for suicide
2. To gain attention
3. To request a particular place for burial
4. To ease the pain of loved ones
5. To increase the pain and guilt of the survivors by placing blame

The expression of hopelessness and the relief from intolerable suffering as a reason for suicide is a common theme. Virginia Woolf, who died March 28, 1941, aged fifty-nine when she drowned herself in the river Ouse near her home, wrote the following letter to her husband Leonard: "Dearest, I feel certain I am going mad again. I feel we can't go through another of those terrible times. And I shan't recover this time. I begin to hear voices, and I can't concentrate. So I am doing what seems the best thing to do. You have given me the greatest possible happiness. You have been in every way all that anyone could be. I don't think two people could have been happier till this terrible disease came. I can't fight any longer" (Szasz 2006, 84).

James Whale, a film director, best known for his work in the 1903 horror movie classics such as *Frankenstein*, *Bride of Frankenstein*, and *The Invisible Man* drowned himself on May 29, 1957, after a long bout of depression. Ironically he left the book *Don't Go Near the Water* by William Brinkley on his bedside table together with a note that read, "The future is just old age and illness and pain.... I must have peace and this is the only way" (Rodriguez 2006, 288).

The author Charlotte Perkins Gilman, who died on August 17, 1935, after a long battle with depression following her developing breast cancer, wrote, "When all usefulness is over, when one is assured of an unavoidable and imminent death, it is the simplest of human rights to choose a quick and easy death in place of a slow and horrible one" (Waithe 1994, 66).

Attempting to ease the pain of others or feeling that the world will be a better place without them is also common. Kurt Cobain was the lead musician of Nirvana, a multi-platinum-selling grunge band that revolutionized the sound of the nineties. Given the sudden and completely unexpected success of the band, the extremely sensitive Cobain turned in part to heroin use in the early 1990s. On March 4, 1994, he was rushed to hospital in a coma after an unsuccessful suicide attempt on prescription painkillers with champagne. After the discharge from the hospital, still depressed, he was encouraged to enter a drug detox program in Los Angeles. Sadly, he remained there for only a few days and then discharged himself. He returned to his house, and, on April 5, 1994, he shot himself. His note read, "Frances and Courtney, I'll be at your altar. Please keep going Courtney, for Frances for her life will be so much happier without me. I LOVE YOU. I LOVE YOU" (Stanton 2003, 48).

Author Hunter Thompson, best known for his book *Fear and Loathing in Las Vegas*, shot himself on February 20, 2005, at the age of sixty-seven after weeks of pain from physical problems that included a broken leg and a hip replacement. He also had not produced any significant literature in more than thirty years. In his note entitled "Football Season Is Over," he wrote, "No More Games. No More Bombs. No More Walking. No More Fun. No More Swimming. 67. That is 17 years past 50. 17 more than I needed or wanted. Boring. I am always bitchy. No Fun for anybody. 67. You are getting Greedy. Act your old age. Relax. This won't hurt" (Vaughn 2007, 42).

Although suicide is the most tragic complication of depression, it need not be the final outcome. Finding a reason, any reason, to keep going is the task of the sufferer and those who love them. Novelist Kurt Vonnegut suffered from terrible depression and attempted suicide in 1984. He was honest about his struggle and, in 2005, told an interviewer, "My father, like Hemingway, was a gun nut and was very unhappy late in life. But he was proud of not commit-ting suicide. And I'll do the same, so as not to set a bad example for my chil-dren." Suicide is certainly the most devastating complication of depression, but it is not the only one. Next we see the economic impact of clinical depres-sion on individuals and society.

ECONOMIC IMPACT

Depression can so totally take over a person's life that all aspects of their life, including their employment, are impacted. Michael was a thirty-six-year-old book editor who presented to the clinic after he had received a perform-ance evaluation saying that he had the lowest productivity in his division. He admitted that he had been suffering from depression but that he had been afraid to mention it to his human resources department for fear that he would lose his job. He said that if he were seen as depressed, this would limit how much his company would invest in him and would diminish any possibility for advancement. He acknowledged that the stress and embarrassment of his con-dition left him feeling profound shame.

The fear of losing a job and the respect of colleagues is often enough to prevent a person from seeking treatment. The consequence of this fear and the ensuing depression can lead to lower productivity and lost worked days. The economic impact to society of depression has been calculated. Walter Stewart, Ph.D., and colleagues (Stewart et al. 2003) conducted research that showed that clinical depression costs the United States about $44 billion annually, including $24 billion from absenteeism and lost productivity. This amount of money would be staggering if it were accurate, but newer research by Dr. Philip Wang, M.D., at Harvard (Wang et al. 2004) shows that previous studies significantly underestimate the adverse economic effects associated with depression!

The treatment of depression would go a long way to stemming such costs. In their study, Wang and colleagues showed that the losses related to depres-sion in the workplace exceeded the costs of effective treatment. However, effective treatment requires effective assessment, and, not only do employees like Michael often avoid seeking treatment, but many employers do not have the resources to recognize the signs of depression in their employees. Many depressed employees believe they can handle their illness on their own. Depressed employees are also often reluctant to ask for help from their com-pany, fearing that their information will not be kept private. Furthermore, given the pharmaceutical and therapy costs of treatment, many smaller self-insured businesses are reluctant to incur such costs.

For the individual, the economic impact of depression is compounded depending on the age of onset of depression. Ernst Berndt, Ph.D., and colleagues (Berndt et al. 2000) looked at the impact of early-onset depression. Specifically, they looked at the onset of depression before age twenty-two and found that early-onset major depressive disorder adversely affected the educational attainment of women but not of men. They found that a randomly selected twenty-one-year-old woman with early-onset depression could expect future annual earnings that were 12–18 percent lower than those of a randomly selected twenty-one-year-old woman whose onset of major depressive disorder occurred after age twenty-one.

Another aspect on the impact of depression on the workplace is the issue of gender. Dr. John Rush, M.D., a psychiatrist at the University of Texas Southwestern Medical Center at Dallas has conducted research that found that more than 9 percent of the U.S. workforce had some kind of depression during any given two-week period and that, because depression is more common in women, businesses with more female employees would be disproportionately affected. He argued that the issue was not as much a business problem as a national issue, requiring the attention of policymakers and healthcare providers.

THE EFFECTS OF DEPRESSION ON PHYSICAL HEALTH

In Chapter 3, we saw how medical illness can cause major depression. Depression, however, can impact the course of medical illness. For instance, in the elderly or in people with serious illness, the presence of depression reduces their survival rates when compared with people with the same illness but without depression. Earlier we saw how depression causes (and is caused by) low serotonin levels. Low serotonin levels in turn lead to stress-related responses in the body that cause inflammation, blood-clotting problems, and in turn damage to cells. When such damage accumulates, it causes damage to whole organs. Fighting the original medical illness becomes all that more difficult. Another issue in depressed people with medical illness is that the low energy state and isolation of depression leads to reduced physical activity and diminished social interactions, which in themselves lead to increased illness severity.

Depression has been shown to increase the incidence and severity of heart attacks, stroke, and death after these events. One of the best-known studies in all of medicine is the Framingham Heart Study. In the late 1950s, more than 5,000 inhabitants of Framingham, Massachusetts, were enrolled in the study. In the 1970s, the children of the original study group were also enrolled in the study. Tremendous research was produced and continues to be produced from this population sample. Researchers knew that stroke caused depression in many patients, but they wanted to see whether there was an association between depression and stroke when the depression occurred before the stroke. Kimberly Salaycik and colleagues (Salaycik, Kelly-Hayes, and Beiser 2007) at Boston University studied 4,000 people aged 29–100 and followed them for up to eight years. They found that people under age sixty-five with a history of depression were more than four times as likely to have a stroke or a transient ischemic attack, which is an episode of low blood flow to the brain, in the next eight years as people under age sixty-five without depression. The researchers suggested that depression might lead to poor adherence to pre-scribed drugs, inadequate diet, or poor physical activity, which in turn caused the problems of low serotonin as described earlier.

Stroke and heart problems are dramatic consequences of depression. Other significant effects of depression, which take a serious toll on physical health, include the following.

1. Obesity: Both obesity and depression are increasing in Americans. Studies show that people who are depressed are at much higher risk of obesity. Studies also show that obese people are more likely than non-obese people to become depressed. Low physical activity in depressed people and the side effects of some of the medications used to treat depression are possible factors in the link between depression and obesity.
2. Increasing sensations of pain: Depression has been shown to increase pain and the experience of pain in people with conditions such as arthritis.
3. Cancer: Depression has a profound impact on quality of life in cancer patients. Research shows that there is a worse outlook in cancer patients with a history of depression but not in patients whose depression occurred after the cancer.
4. Alcohol, smoking, and drug abuse: Research shows that about 14 percent of people with major depression also abuse alcohol, that 26 percent of people with major depression are nicotine dependent, and that 5 percent have drug abuse problems. It is often considered that people who suffer from depression turn to alcohol, nicotine, and drugs to medicate themselves.

STIGMA

Stigma: (n.) a mark of disgrace or infamy; a stain or reproach, as on one's reputation.

"The last great stigma of the twentieth century is the stigma of mental illness": so said Tipper Gore in June 1999 at the first White House conference on mental health. Distrust, stereotyping, fear, embarrassment, and anger manifest the stigmatization of people with mental disorders. The stigma leads others to avoid socializing or working with, renting to, or employing people with mental disorders. Sadly, this has been true for as long as people have suffered from mental illness. The history of the treatment of the mentally ill is a history filled with many accounts of neglect, cruelty, and maltreatment. In the middle ages, possession by evil spirits, moral weakness, and other such explanations stigmatized the mentally ill. Often, the responsibility for a cure was placed on the patients themselves. Those who weren't cured were chained to walls in institutions such as the infamous Bedlam, where the rest of society could forget that they had ever existed.

Conditions in these institutions were inhumane. Patients were crammed into dark, musty cells and were at times chained to their beds. There was no fresh air, no light, and poor food, and the punishment for misbehavior was a severe beating. There are accounts of women being committed for attempting to leave their husband because, clearly, an evil spirit was inducing them to commit adultery.

The mentally ill were stigmatized in the middle ages, and so they are today. Football great Terry Bradshaw, who himself suffered from severe depression, noted this when he said, "Stigma is incredibly powerful. We'll talk about cancer and every other disease, including alcohol and drug abuse, but people do not want to talk about depression. There's something about depression that seems to say, 'I'm a tremendous failure' or 'I'm the biggest wuss there is'" (Morgan 2004).

The symptoms of depression are hardly symptoms that a person would willingly choose, yet, sadly, many people view depression as a character flaw. One study by the National Mental Health Association reported that 54 percent of people believe depression is a personal weakness. In England, the nature of the stigma of depression was captured by how professional soccer player Stan Collymore, who played for the English national team, was treated. He developed a severe depression, and his career went into a rapid decline. Collymore also played for the professional team Aston Villa. In interviews, he has said that he found it hard to forgive how his team manager reacted to his depression. Collymore recalls the manager as saying that Collymore had to "pull his socks up" and that the manager's idea of depression was "that of a woman living on a 20th floor apartment with kids." *The Sun* newspaper's sports writers compounded the stigmatization of depression when they wrote that Collymore should be kicked out of soccer because how could anyone be depressed when he is "earning so much money." William Styron, the author of *Darkness Visible*, a memoir of his struggle with depression, once said, "the pain of severe depression is quite unimaginable to those who have not suffered it" (Styron 1990, 33).

Research on the effects of stigma in the mentally ill varies, with some reports finding that as many as 70 percent reported discrimination. Other reports have shown that, although many patients report feeling stigmatized by their illness, their communities are in fact supportive of the mentally ill and that discrimination occurs less than perceived. Interestingly, although perhaps not surprisingly, a study (Perlick et al. 2001) found that people felt more stigmatized during the active or acute phase of their illness (for example, during hospitalization for depression) and that the more they were concerned about the stigma of the depression, the worse they did socially after being discharged from the hospital. Clearly, it is not only the stigma but the perception of the stigma as well as when in their illness they feel stigmatized that can have a profound impact on a person's well being.

Despite the fact that the mentally ill are no longer accused of having succumbed to spells, incantations, or of having committed adultery and they are no longer chained to walls or crammed into tiny cells, the inconsiderate views of prominent people can rapidly spread through the media, and humiliate a sufferer. TV chat-show host Rosie O'Donnell and real estate tycoon Donald Trump have had a war of words for years. She has insulted him on TV, and he has retaliated in the press. Many think, however, that he crossed the line when, after she announced on her show *The View* that she has been treated for depression, he made a statement on *Entertainment Tonight*: "I have no compassion for Rosie.... I can fully understand that when she looks in the mirror she suffers from depression."

Some of the reasons for this stigma include the lack of a definitive test, such as an x-ray or a blood test that shows depression. It is as if somebody with a broken bone or a large surgical scar visually appears more legitimately ill. At times, people are judged for their "reasons" for being depressed or are seen as making depression to be a convenient excuse for not having to do something.

President Ford's wife, Betty Ford, admitted to depression, cancer, alcoholism, and addiction thirty years ago at a time when the stigma of these illnesses was far greater than it is today, and yet today, even doctors collude with patients around hiding the truth. Most famously, NBC's Jane Pauley went public with her manic depression in 2006, although her doctor had recommended that she tell NBC she had a thyroid condition rather than her mental illness!

Because many people with depression fear that they will be labeled as being mentally ill, they do not seek treatment. This stigma even extends to some doctors and politicians, who may be less willing to support programs and policies that would improve mental-health care, and yet depression will strike doctors and politicians just the same. "We're not ashamed of it. Depression is something a lot of people suffer from," said Deval Patrick, governor of Massachusetts, on acknowledging that his wife suffers from depression (as quoted in the *Boston Globe*).

It helps the cause of mental illnesses such as depression when public officials can readily acknowledge the condition, but at times, this is not the case. For instance, in Australia, a federal official was challenged on an Australian government proposal that people who were suffering from depression after an injury would no longer be able to sue for being depressed. The official responded, "What that is directed to, is to ensure that those who do have a recognized mental illness are compensated. But people who might be just malingering, if you like, or just have an anxiety condition or depression that they really do need to get over and get back to work—well obviously they're not going to be compensated just to stay out of the workforce." The implication was that depression was merely an optional condition and that physical illness secondary to an injury was somehow more legitimate.

As a general rule, people find it much easier to talk about a physical complaint than an emotional one (which is one of the reasons that many people don't seek help for mental illnesses). It is as if the physical symptom or problem "happened" to them and so they are not at "fault," whereas an emotional problem is sometimes seen as a weakness that can simply be overcome and if not implies some serious intrinsic flaw in the person. Furthermore, many people can find it "uncomfortable" to be around a person who is upset. It embarrasses them because they don't know what to say to help them or it embarrasses them that the person is making a scene, which somehow reflects on the person trying to help.

Stigma can affect people directly such as a refusal to hire the person, communally as there are often fewer resources for treatment, and individually as these effects begin to take a toll on a person's self-esteem. Sadly, a tragic consequence of the stigma of mental illness is that it can engender a significant loss of self-esteem because the sufferer concludes that he or she is a failure or that they have little of which to be proud. One study (Link et al. 2001) looked at the effect of stigma on seventy mentally ill people on their self-esteem. In the study, the researchers looked at how the mentally ill perceived rejection and discrimination and found that, the more a mentally ill person felt that they had been discriminated against, the worse their self-esteem. The take-home point was that reducing stigma would have the added benefit of improving self-esteem in the psychiatrically ill.

However, all the work in the community can be dealt a serious blow by the actions of a high-profile celebrity, like when actor Tom Cruise disparaged the treatment of depression. He slammed actress Brooke Shields for the fact that she used the antidepressant Paxil when she suffered from severe postpartum depression following the birth of her baby. He said that there was "no science behind" antidepressant use, that they are dangerous, and that she could have recovered using just vitamins. Without equal access to the media, such a statement would have remained unchallenged, but Brooke Shields came back and said, "I'm going to take a wild guess and say that Mr. Cruise has never suffered from postpartum depression." She continued her crusade and went on to write a *New York Times* Op/Ed piece in which she stated, "comments like those made by Tom Cruise are a disservice to mothers everywhere. To suggest that I was wrong to take drugs to deal with my depression, and that instead I should have taken vitamins and exercised shows an utter lack of understanding about postpartum depression and childbirth in general.... If any good can come of Mr. Cruise's ridiculous rant, let's hope that it gives much-needed attention to a serious disease. Perhaps now is the time to call on doctors, particularly obstetricians and pediatricians, to screen for postpartum depression. After all, during the first three months after childbirth, you see a pediatrician at least three times. While pediatricians are trained to take care of children, it would make sense for them to talk with new mothers, ask questions and inform them of the symptoms and treatment should they show signs of postpartum depression."

Although Brooke Shields's postpartum depression became the stuff of tabloids, perhaps no other pregnancy-related depression has had more scrutiny than that of Crown Princess Masako, the wife of Crown Prince Naruhito of Japan. Princess Masako is a Harvard-educated former diplomat, who had hoped to bring the Japanese Crown into the twenty-first century with the promise of a contemporary woman in the Royal Palace. However, once married, she was under tremendous pressure to perform a single duty, and that was to "produce" a male heir. After years of fertility treatment, she finally had a daughter, Princess Aiko. The Imperial Household Agency, which is the powerful bureaucracy that oversees the royal family, pressured Masako to have another child. The matter was so serious that the then prime minister, Junichiro Koizumi, gathered a group of experts that recommended that a woman and her offspring be allowed to ascend the throne. This recommendation brought tremendous resistance from Japanese conservatives, who insisted that a male only could ascend to the throne. Furthermore, Prince Tomohito, a cousin of the emperor, argued for the revival of the concubine system, which historically provided that plenty of child-bearing women be available to the emperor. Under the weight of the scrutiny of her private and personal life, Princess Masako eventually slipped into a depression. Her depression led the crown prince to hold an unprecedented news conference, in which he stated that he would not let his wife be sacrificed for the greater good of the monarchy.

The clash of culture versus individual dignity had come to a head.

Nearly four years after her "failure" to have a boy child, the pressure on the princess lifted a little when Princess Kiko, the wife of the emperor's younger son, gave birth to a boy, securing the succession to the imperial throne for another generation. Masako's depression appeared to lift and, after years in the seclusion of the royal palace, she started to once again appear in public. Sadly, neither Emperor Akihito nor palace officials ever acknowledged the problem publicly, once again adding to the stigma of mental illness. Had the depression received official exposure, it would have exposed the fact that at least one in five people in Japan suffer from a mental illness. The effect would have been similar to that of the highly publicized death from cancer of politician Shintaro Abe, who was the father of a former prime minister. Until his death, cancer was rarely ever talked about publicly or reported in the press as a cause of death!

A very different approach to a high-profile depression occurred in early 2007 when, after having labored exhaustively as her husband Deval Patrick's major supporter in their successful bid for the Massachusetts Governorship, first lady Diane Patrick succumbed to depression. The official public announcement read, "First Lady Diane Patrick is being treated for exhaustion and depression. The governor will work a flexible schedule for the next few weeks in order to spend more time with her and his family. The family asks for the prayers and understanding of the public."

It was not only the sudden thrust into a public spotlight after unrelenting campaigning but the demands of her new office, as well as trying to balance this with her own professional life as a top partner in a prestigious law firm and personal life as wife and mother to two daughters, that led to her depression. The stigma of depression cuts across all social classes and cultures. Despite the vast numbers of people who suffer from mental illness, it is often more accepted and less stigmatizing to have a physical illness than a mental one.

I remember as a resident in psychiatry being asked to evaluate a middle-aged man who had been suffering from a low-grade depression for years. It had now reached the point that he had begun to experience suicidal thoughts. I asked him why he had not sought treatment earlier. He answered, "I regret not doing so. So many people at work talk about people with mental illness as if they are crazy. I thought that I am going to be labeled nutcase, or crazy.

I would be one of *them*, the ones my colleagues talked about. I wasn't willing to go through that. I wished that I had had a thyroid problem or something."

Education and acknowledgment of the problem are essential to address the stigma. As Amy Tan, the best-selling author of the *Joy Luck Club* who suffered from depression said in a 1995 interview, "People look at me as this very, I don't know, Confucius-like wise person—which I'm not. They don't see all the shit that I've been through. And going back to the question of being a role model, well, my life hasn't been perfect. I needed help" (www.salon.com).

IMPACT ON THE FAMILY

Julie Totten founded Families for Depression Awareness (http://familyaware. org) after sensing that something was wrong with her brother but wasn't sure what it was. He had complained of many of the physical manifestations of major depression—headaches, stomach upset, and fatigue—but did not discuss his symptoms with anyone, and, suffering from depression, tragically, he committed suicide at the age of twenty-six.

Totten has pointed out that, although depression is typically considered to be a mental illness that affects an individual, it should more accurately be considered as a family illness, one that requires support from parents and siblings.

Depression in an individual can have a profound impact not only on their own lives but also on the lives of their families and the people who love them.

Effects of Depression on a Marriage

Depression's cruelest trick is eroding love until even its memories fade and, like faces in old photographs, no longer seem familiar.

(Sheffield 2003)

Jillian was a thirty-two-year-old mother of a six-month-old child who been married to her husband for the past two and a half years, although they had dated for three years before they were married. She was becoming increasingly concerned because, soon after they married, he had become increasingly depressed and that in part it had to do with a demanding job that kept him away from home three or four days a week due to travel. Jillian felt that she too was becoming depressed and was having a hard time dealing after the birth of the baby but that she did not want to ask her husband for help because of his depression. Despite her feeling that they had been in love when they met, she was worried that her relationship was in serious trouble. Sadly, many couples suffer when one in the family has depression.

Research shows that, when one spouse suffers from depression, both will have an unhappy marriage (Whisman, Uebelacker, and Weinstock 2004). His research shows that being in a relationship with someone with mental health problems may lower the satisfaction for the partner. The burden of living with someone who has mental health problems takes a toll.

In their study, Whisman and colleagues recruited 774 married couples from seven states. Each partner was tested for depression, anxiety, and whether they had a happy or unhappy marriage. They found that, if a spouse had high levels of anxiety and depression, that this predicted an unhappy marriage not only for the depressed spouse but for the other spouse as well.

The more anxious and/or depressed either spouse was, the more dissatisfied he or she was with the marriage. Another important finding was that depression (more than anxiety) affected whether a person considered himself or herself to be in a happy or unhappy marriage. The recommendation was made that, when treating spouses with an unhappy marriage, therapists should closely evaluate each of the partners' mental health.

The evaluation, however, doesn't end there. For many families, children are significantly impacted by a parent's depression.

When a Parent Is Depressed

Eliza was a thirteen-year-old girl who presented to the clinic brought in by her mother, who said that Eliza's grades had been steadily falling over the past six months and that Eliza had admitted to her that she had smoked marijuana the weekend prior to her evaluation. Her mother was extremely worried over the rapid decline given that Eliza had been near the top of her class. Her mother admitted that her daughter's rapid deterioration began soon after her husband James (Eliza's father) had been hospitalized for treatment of severe depression and suicidal thinking.

In his book *Undoing Depression: What Therapy Doesn't Teach You and Medication Can't Give You and Active Treatment of Depression*, psychologist Richard O'Connor states that there is much research showing that children of depressed parents are themselves at high risk for depression, substance abuse, and antisocial activities (O'Connor 1997).

It is certainly evident in even much younger children; studies have found that depressed mothers have difficulty bonding with their infants, are less sensitive to the baby's needs, and less consistent in their responses to the baby's behavior. The babies of depressed mothers appear more unhappy than babies of mothers who are not depressed. The babies of depressed mothers tend to be more difficult to comfort, be more difficult to feed and put to sleep. When they reach the toddler stage, the kids of depressed mothers tend to be more difficult to handle, more defiant, and generally more negative.

These traits in a child often make the role of parenting much more difficult and can reinforce the parent's sense that they are a failure and worthless. A parent refusing to get treatment makes the outlook bad for the child. The child can grow up believing they are unlovable, to blame for their parent's depression, and an inconvenience. Unable to self-soothe, they are at risk for substance abuse, not knowing how to ask for help they can be disruptive, feeling unworthy as a child they are at risk for depression, and without knowing how to fit in they are at risk for social isolation.

Dr. William R. Beardslee, M.D., is the Academic Chairman of Psychiatry at Children's Hospital Boston and author of *Out of the Darkened Room—When a Parent Is Depressed: Protecting the Children and Strengthening the Family* (Beardslee 2002). He is another expert who has written extensively on the effect of a parent's depression on their child.

Beardslee has pointed out that a big issue when a parent has depression is the family not talking, or at least not talking enough with their children about the depression. His research has shown that, even in families who talk about most things openly, being open about depression is difficult in large part because the parent who is depressed feels so bad and often blames himself or herself. Furthermore, because depression can appear in so many different ways, including behaviors such as withdrawal and irritability, this can lead to confusion and fear in children, making communication difficult.

He recommends first having a conversation with the nondepressed spouse and then with the children and that the focus ought to be on the promise of treatment and hope for the future. One specific suggestion is to tell family stories that highlight the positive in the family.

The Effect of a Child's Depression on a Family

Parents often have a difficult time recognizing depression in their adolescents due to the common developmental withdrawal of an adolescent from their family. Conversely, teens with depression don't tend to pull away as much from their friends as adults with depression do from their social situations. Teens may socialize less, but they usually don't give up their friendships. We often have the situation that a parent finds out about their child's depression because the child's friend has informed the parent. By the time a teen has disconnected from his or her friends, the depression is significant and has been going on a long time. It is a common finding that depressed children have depressed parents. It is possible that this is pure genetics at play, but there are often difficult circumstances at play, such as conflict, domestic violence, poverty, or alcoholism, which can lead to poor parenting. Furthermore, a depressed, hyperactive child can be hard to raise. When the decision to get treatment for the child is finally made, the stress of having a depressed child is compounded by having to take time off work to make therapy or hospital appointments. Parents also often have to make the hard decision of choosing whether to place their child on medications and, if so, which one to chose.

Whether depression leads to suicide, stroke, worsening isolation, economic distress, or stigma, clearly treating the condition as early and as aggressively as possible is essential. If there is any hope to reduce these devastating complications, research needs to continue. The future does, however, look promising, and we examine this promise in the next chapter.

6

Depression: The Future

The best thing about the future is that it comes only one day at a time.
(Abraham Lincoln, quoted in Pine 2002, 42)

In the year 2253, some twelve years before he signed aboard with Captain Kirk (the commander of the Starship Enterprise), Dr. "Bones" McCoy had developed a neural grafting procedure using the creation of nerve pathways between the graft and a patient's basal ganglia, a procedure that would still be in practice over a century later. In the popular *Star Trek* series, the fictional Dr. McCoy needed simply to wave his tricorder sensor over ailing crewmembers to detect any illness and to cure many of them by this simple act. In the era before the Starship Enterprise had counselors, he was the psychologist especially for the ship's two senior officers.

Tricorders and neural grafting may be a thing of the future but perhaps not too distant a future. Over recent years, radical new ideas have changed the way we think about the brain and how we view and treat depression.

BACTERIA TO TREAT DEPRESSION?

Many of the current medication strategies for treating depression aim to increase the amount of serotonin in the brain. We know that some bacteria cause disease, but the idea that bacteria may prevent disease is not something that people generally consider. There is, however, some evidence that exposure to bacteria may in fact relieve the symptoms of clinical depression by increasing serotonin levels. As sometimes happens with such discoveries, this one too was a chance observation.

Dr. Mary O'Brien, M.D., an oncologist at the Royal Marsden Hospital in London, was trying an experimental treatment for lung cancer that involved infecting patients with a bacterium known as *Mycobacterium vaccae*. This bacterium is a harmless relative of the bugs that cause tuberculosis and leprosy and is commonly found in soil. Other than the finding that her patients had fewer symptoms of the cancer, she also noted an improvement in their overall happiness!

To explain why the patients felt better, Dr. Chris Lowry, Ph.D. (Lowry et al. 2007), a neuroscientist at Bristol University, and his colleagues proposed the

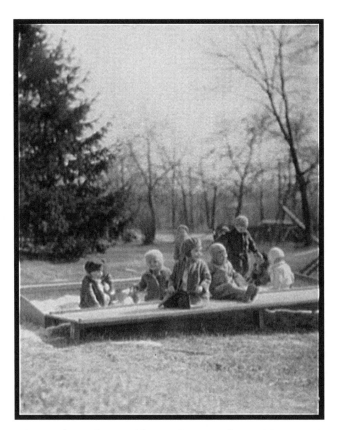

Figure 6.1. Getting down, dirty, and happy. *Courtesy Library of Congress, Prints & Photographs Division, Theodor Horydczak Collection, LC-H813-1290-003.*

following theory. They suggested that *Mycobacterium vaccae* caused the brain to produce serotonin. To prove their theory, they infected mice with this *Mycobacterium*. This appeared to alter the mouse behavior in ways similar to that produced by giving mice antidepressant drugs. The mice appeared to be much more stress free than the untreated mice. Studying the mice brains, those treated with the bacteria in fact had produced more serotonin.

Over the years, researchers have wondered why the rates of depression appear to be going up, together with the rates of asthma and allergies. One idea is that, as parents become more vigilant about dirt and hygiene, children have become less exposed to all kinds of bugs, including the harmless ones. This lack of exposure to bugs, both good and bad, has weakened our immune system because the immune system needs foreign invaders to be strong and active. Allowing children to get down and dirty in the play yard might be one long-term preventative measure for depression. Furthermore, another possibility is that perhaps clinical depression could be treated with a vaccination. A patient would go in and get a flu shot and perhaps their *Mycobacterium vaccae* antidepression vaccine!

SEARCHING FOR THE HOLY GRAIL OF DEPRESSION: A COMMON BRAIN PATHWAY

One of the unanswered questions of depression is how there can be so many different causes and so many different treatments that seem to work. Finding a common brain pathway for all of these would go a long way to answering this question. Researchers at Stanford University (Airan et al. 2007) are closing in on finding such a pathway.

The researchers created animal models of depression in rats and then treated the rats with antidepressants. They found that the differing mechanisms of depression and treatments appeared to funnel through a single brain circuit. They found common brain activity in all their rats in a part of the hippocampus known as the dentate gyrus. The dentate gyrus has historically been considered a part of the brain crucial for encoding new information and new memories. It is also one of the few places in the adult brain where the growth of new brain cells takes place. In the research, the rats that had depression had decreased activity in the dentate gyrus. The activity then increased when the rats were treated with antidepressants.

The Stanford findings supported prior research that had shown that growth of new brain cells (a process called neurogenesis) in the dentate gyrus was necessary for antidepressants to cure rats of their depression. In the Stanford study, when the depressed rats were fed fluoxetine (the generic name for

Prozac), they experienced rapid neurogenesis and the same electrical activity in their dentate gyri as normal rats.

If these findings are found to be true or similar in humans as well, targeting the dentate gyrus may be the key in the treatment of depression.

STEM CELLS AS A CURE?

Stem cells are cells found in all multicellular organisms that retain the ability to renew themselves and, under specific influences, can go on to become the cells of any organ in the body. This ability holds tremendous promise for people who, for example, might need a new heart or new serotonin-producing nerve cells, because these could in theory be grown from these stem cells.

Although the use of embryonic stem cells (those are stem cells found in human embryos) remains a very controversial and political issue in the United States, scientists around the world have eagerly embraced the practice. Multiple sclerosis (MS) is a chronic, inflammatory disease that leads to the loss of myelin, the protective covering of nerve cells in the brain. This can cause a variety of symptoms, including changes in sensation, visual problems, muscle weakness, depression, difficulties with coordination and speech, severe fatigue, problems with balance, and pain.

In a report from Ukraine on the use of stem cells in MS, the researchers used embryonic stem cells in twenty-four patients. They found that 70 percent of the patients got better. They found that those who showed improvement had decreased weakness, improved appetite and mood, and decreased depression.

This research will need to be repeated by other researchers if the results are to be considered valid, but there is no reason to imagine that stem cells will not play a part in the treatment of depression and other neurological illnesses in the future.

A GENE FOR MAJOR DEPRESSION AND A POSSIBLE CURE?

There is a biological reaction called "apoptosis," that is a process involving a genetically programmed series of events leading to the death of a cell.

In 2006, a Salt Lake City-based company, Myriad Genetics, announced that it had discovered a gene known as the "Apoptosis Protease Activating Factor 1" (or Apaf-1) gene that causes major depression. The Apaf-1 gene was discovered using large families from Utah that had multiple cases of major depressive disorder.

The Apaf-1 gene makes a protein known (not surprisingly) as the Apaf-1 protein. This protein then causes a series of chemical reactions that lead ultimately to destruction of a cell. The hypothesis is that it is this cell death or cell destruction that leads to depression in these families.

The discovery has important implications for the development of a new class of medications to treat depression. The idea would be to create a drug that blocks the action of the Apaf-1 protein. This in turn would stop the protein from killing brain cells and conceivably lead to less depression.

GENES THAT PREDICT ANTIDEPRESSANT RESPONSE

In a study by the NIMH researchers (Paddock et al. 2007) found that variation in a gene called GRIK4 (glutamate receptor, ionotropic, kainate 4) appears to make people with depression more likely to respond to the medication citalopram (commercially known as Celexa) than people who do not have the GRIK4 variation. The increased likelihood of response to Celexa was small. However, the researchers had found a year earlier that patients with the variation of a gene known as HTR2A (5-hydroxytryptamine receptor 2A) also had a small increase in the likelihood to respond to Celexa.

A much more powerful finding was that people who had both of the variations, that is those who had GRIK4 and HTR2A, were 23 percent more likely to respond to citalopram than were people with neither variation.

This finding hints strongly at the possibility that the differences in patient's response to antidepressant medications are based partly on gene differences. Genetic studies may lead to a better understanding of which treatments are likely to work for each patient, and, in the future, medication treatment choices might routinely be preceded by genetic testing.

SMALL SWITCHES THAT TURN BRAIN CELLS ON AND OFF

One of the foremost researchers in brain function is psychiatrist Dr. Karl Deisseroth at Stanford University. His particular area of interest includes brain circuits as they pertain to depression. He has noted that intensive treatments, such as ECT, can effectively cure depression but often with side effects such as memory loss and headaches. Deisseroth is also a bioengineer, and he has developed a new method for controlling the activity of brain cells with flashes of light. It is a technology that could one day lead to more precise and safer targeted treatments for psychiatric disorders such as depression.

He has argued that brains are intricate, electrical structures, so that it is far too simplistic to describe mental illness as a chemical imbalance. He likes to think of the brain in terms of circuits. "Talking to a patient that's depressed," he says, "you get a sense that [brain] activity is not flowing appropriately."

His thinking was that, to identify the circuits of depression, he had to be able to turn brain circuits on and off to see what these circuits did. The usual way to turn brain cell circuits on and off is with electrodes that activate neurons with jolts of electricity. This method is however not precise enough, so he and fellow researchers developed another technique.

Deisseroth and his colleagues used a protein obtained from green algae to act as an "on switch." They then genetically engineered neurons that could produce that algae protein. Then, when the neuron was exposed to light, the protein would turn on and cause electrical activity within the cell. This electrical activity would then be spread to all the other nerve cells in the brain circuit. This electrical activity could then easily be picked up by sensors and the researchers would see what the response of triggering that specific circuit was, for instance, the twitch of a muscle or the release of a brain chemical.

Deisseroth is using this genetic light switch to study the biological basis of depression. He took a group of rats that showed symptoms similar to those seen in depressed humans. His researchers inserted the protein switch into nerve cells in the different parts of the brain that are linked to depression. They then shone a tiny light onto those nerve cells to look for circuits that lead to improvement of symptoms. By finding those circuits, Deisseroth believes that scientists could develop more targeted antidepressants.

Deisseroth has said, "Prozac goes to all the circuits in the brain, rather than just the relevant ones. That's part of the reason it has so many side effects."

Eventually, the goal of this therapy is that, by targeting specific nerve cells, more exact treatments with fewer side effects will evolve.

CONCLUSION

"I have deep feelings of depression," Charlie Brown said to Lucy in an early Peanuts strip. "What can I do about it?"

"Snap out if it," advised Lucy.

Were it only that easy. The sentiments expressed by the fictional Charlie Brown are only too real for a large proportion of the world, and the number of people suffering from depression is growing.

Studies suggest that rates of major depression are increasing and that the age of onset of depression is decreasing. In fact, there has been an increase in the rates of depression for all ages. Despite the increase in overall depression, some statistics remain the same, such as the persistent gender difference with the risk of depression consistently two to three times higher in women than in men across all adult ages, and a persistent family effect, with the risk of having depression being about two to three times higher in people who have first-degree relatives who suffer from depression.

The toll that the illness will take on individuals, families, and society is hardly measurable. One thing that is clear is that, as the world has become technologically more complex, the number of people suffering from depression has increased. Perhaps, however, technology will in turn provide the answers, and Doctor McCoy's tricorder and Lucy's advice will be just the thing to treat depression.

Timeline

Remember that there is nothing stable in human affairs; therefore avoid undue elation in prosperity, or undue depression in adversity.

(Socrates)

5000 BC   The practice of drilling a hole in the skull, known as trepanation, is used to release evil spirits believed to be responsible for madness.

1500 BC   The Ebers Papyrus, the most important of the ancient medical papyri, contains a description of clinical depression with incantations to be used to turn away the evil spirits thought to cause depression.

550 BC   Probably the oldest subjective description of clinical depression ever written, taken from the Book of Psalms 6:6–7, was by the biblical King David: "I am worn out from groaning; all night long I flood my bed with weeping and drench my couch with tears. My eyes grow weak with sorrow; they fail because of all my foes." There are multiple biblical references to depression and even to suicide following depression. The book of Samuel tells of the depression of King Saul who is tormented by the affliction, and then later, when he is overwhelmed by the prospect of his battle against the Philistines, he asks an armor bearer to kill him. The armor bearer refuses, so Saul takes his own life.

400 BC   Hippocrates, a Greek physician, is considered to be the father of modern medicine. He recognized that ill health had a physical explanation and was not caused by evil spirits, which was the prevailing theory of his day and parenthetically remains the belief in many cultures around the world today. His theory was that the body contained four bodily fluids or humors. The humors were phlegm, blood, black bile, and yellow bile. Illness came from a disturbance in the balance of any of the humors. The view of depression, or melancholia as it was known, was that there was an excess of black bile within the body. The word melancholia is a derivation of the Greek words for black (melas) and bile (khole).

45–125 AD   Mestrius Plutarch, the Greek philosopher, wrote the following clear description about depression: "Every little evil is magnified by the scaring specters of his anxiety. He looks on himself as a man whom the gods hate and pursue with their anger.... Awake, he makes no use of his reason; and asleep, he enjoys no respite from his alarms. His reason always slumbers; his fears are always awake. Nowhere can he find escape from his imaginary terrors."

170 AD   Galen, a Greek physician, recommended the use of electric eels for treating headaches and facial pain.

200 AD   Aretaeus of Cappodocia, a Greek Physician, was just as descriptive: "And yet in certain of these cases there is mere anger and grief and sad dejection of mind ... those affected with melancholy are not every one of them affected according to one particular form but they are suspicious of poisoning or flee to the desert from misanthropy or turn superstitious or contract a hatred of life. Or if at any time a relaxation takes place, in most cases hilarity supervenes. The patients are dull or stern, dejected or unreasonably torpid ... they also become peevish, dispirited and start up from a disturbed sleep."

1000 AD	Not much headway was made in the understanding or the treatment of depression until the middle ages. The humor theory prevailed together with the strong belief in the influence of evil spirits on the development of mental illness. After becoming a physician at sixteen, the great Islamic philosopher-physician Avicenna wrote on the relationship between the body and soul in a book known as the *Canon of Medicine*. He proposed cures for the mentally ill. His *Canon on Medicine* was so comprehensive that it was still being used in the 1600s.
1400s	In Europe, in the 1400s, there are references to the use of St. John's Wort for the treatment of various maladies, including depression. St. John's Wort continues to be evaluated today for its role in the treatment of depression. Although the first asylums to treat the mentally ill were founded in Europe in the 1400s, casting out evil spirits was still the preferred method for treating mental illness.
1586	English physician Timothie Bright published *Treatise on Melancholy*, the first book written in English on the subject of mental illness, and looked at depression in Elizabethan England. In it, he writes this description of the gloom of depression: "the fancy ouertaken with gastly fumes of melancholy, and the whole force of the spirit closed up in the dungion of melancholy darkness, imagineth all dark, blacke and full of feare."
1599	French Anatomist Andreas Laurentius publishes *A Discourse of the Preservation of the Sight of Melancholike Diseases of Rheumes, and of Old Age*. He wrote, "Melancholike man … is alwaies disquieted both in bodie and spirit, he is subject to watchfulnes, which doth consume him on the one side, and unto sleepe, which tormenteth him on the other side … hee is become a savadge creature, haunting the shadowed places, suspicious, solitarie, enemie to the Sunne, and one whom nothing can please, but onely discontentment, which forgeth unto it selfe a thousand false and vaine imaginations."
1621	Robert Burton published *The Anatomy of Melancholy, What it is: With all the Kinds, Causes, Symptomes, Prognostickes, and Several Cures of it. In Three Maine Partitions with their several Sections,*

Members, and Subsections. Philosophically, Historically, Opened and Cut up. It was an extensive review on the subject of depression, a tome of more than 1,200 pages. He wrote, "This Melancholy of which we are to treat, is a habit, a serious ailment, a settled humour, as Aurelianus and others call it, not errant, but fixed: and as it was long increasing, so, now being (pleasant or painful) grown to a habit, it will hardly be removed." He also noted, "There is no greater cause of melancholy than idleness, no better cure than business." We see that, nearly 2,000 years after Hippocrates, the concept of and reference to the "humor" as a cause of depression remains. Despite great gains in the care of psychiatric patients, there was still little understanding of the underlying causes. Advocates proposed more treatment and less punishment of the mentally ill, and conditions continued to improve for depressed and other mentally ill patients.

1667   French Doctor Jean-Baptiste Denis conducted the first reported use of a blood transfusion to treat depression. The patient suffered from melancholy, and the blood donor was a calf.

1763   A French "nerve doctor" Pierre Pomme, who had been physician to the king, claimed to have discovered the condition, which he named "vapors." Its symptoms are consistent with what we would recognize as depression. He described that such patients suffered with "Fatigue, pain and a sense of dullness." He added that "sadness, melancholy and discouragement poison all of their amusements." His recommended cure was chicken soup and cold baths.

1800s   A theory in the 1800s proposed that you could tell the character of a man, including his psychological makeup and whether he was prone to melancholy, by studying the size, shape, and bumps on his skull. The study of the shape of the head, known as phrenology, had plenty of adherents.

Mid-1800s   The British psychiatrist John Charles Bucknill used electrical stimulation of the skin and potassium oxide to treat patients with melancholic depression, and the use of this new shock therapy remained fairly popular, although controversial, through much of the rest of the century.

1859	Dr. Pablo Mantegazzo isolated cocaine from the coca leaf and wrote about its wonderful powers to combat fatigue, depression, and impotence.
Turn of the twentieth century	Sigmund Freud developed the concept of psychoanalytical therapies or so-called "talk therapies" to treat mental illnesses. This was a major breakthrough in the treatment of depression.
1927	Psychiatrist Dr. Manfred Sakel discovers insulin shock therapy for schizophrenia and other psychiatric disorders.
1934	Ladislas Joseph von Meduna, a Hungarian physician, introduced Metrazol convulsive treatment. Metrazol is a chemical that induces a state of such profound fear that it leads to convulsions. These convulsions were found to be helpful in the treatment of depression, and the drug was widely used in America into the early 1940s.
1935	Egas Moniz performs the first prefrontal lobotomy to treat psychoses. A year later, he published the positive results of his first twenty operations on patients suffering various psychiatric conditions, including anxiety, depression, and schizophrenia.
1936	Neurologist and psychiatrist Walter Freeman performs the first lobotomy in the United States. He would go on to perform 3,439 lobotomies.
1938	Italian neurologist Ugo Cerletti and psychiatrist Lucio Bini recognize the efficacy of convulsive therapy but also the concerning side-effects. They develop electroconvulsive therapy (ECT) and use it for the first time on a human patient.
1940	American psychiatrist Abram Elting Bennett combined metrazol injections with curare, a muscle relaxant, to neutralize the strong muscle contractions.
1950s	The dawn of the development of useful psychiatric medication. Like many drugs, antidepressants were discovered by accident. The first antidepressants discovered in the 1950s belonged to a group of drugs originally developed to treat tuberculosis. The next group was the tricyclic antidepressants, which were developed soon thereafter. These were followed by the development of the so-called selective-serotonin reuptake inhibitors in the

early 1970s and remain the drugs of choice today. The serotonin and norepinephrine reuptake inhibitors are even newer drugs. During the time of drug development, psychiatrists and psychologists began to break away from the orthodoxy of Freud's psychoanalytic theory and practice. Furthermore, many people preferred the idea of psychotherapy or counseling to medication or ECT.

1960s and 1970s   The newer depression-specific psychotherapies, including cognitive-behavioral therapy popularized by Aaron Beck, were introduced.

Late 1970s and 1980s   Gerald Klerman developed interpersonal psychotherapy.

1990s   Marsha Linehan developed dialectical behavioral therapy (DBT) for suicidal patients. DBT has proven to be very effective in reducing suicide and self-destructive behaviors.

2005   An implantable device known as a vagus nerve stimulator is approved for the Food and Drug Administration for the treatment of depression. This device is implanted into a person's chest and delivers mild electrical pulses every five minutes to the vagus nerve, which carries the pulse to the brain.

2006   The discovery is made that variations in the DNA sequence of a gene known as the angiotensin-converting enzyme gene is associated with unipolar depression.

2007   Research shows that cardiac patients struggling with major depression are at double the risk of suffering a heart attack than cardiac patients who are mentally healthy.

2008   A gene is discovered that protects the brain from foreign substances. Researchers find that subtle changes in the gene (known as P-gp) predict the efficacy of two widely used antidepressant drugs. The gene codes for a "transporter" protein that carries antidepressants from the blood into the brain. In some people this transport happens readily, whereas in others it happens very poorly; this is determined by the type of P-gp a person has. The implication is that in the future genetic testing will help determine the type of antidepressant to use, or whether an antidepressant will work at all.

So here we are. What does the future bring? Vaccines against depression? Genetic manipulation of the brain neurons? Stem cell treatments? Brain transplants? All far fetched for now, but the explosive growth of medical discovery is bringing these ideas within the realm of the thinkable and will doubtless extend our timeline as it pertains to depression.

Glossary

Acetylcholine: A neurotransmitter that appears to be involved in learning and memory.

Adrenaline (also known as epinephrine): A hormone that also acts as a neurotransmitter. It is extremely important in the fight-or-flight response, because it signals the heart to pump harder to get ready for action.

Affect: A subjectively experienced feeling state (emotion) and the observable behavior that represents it.

Alexithymia: The inability to describe emotions in a verbal manner.

Allele: An alternate form of a gene. Variations in hair color and other inherited characteristics are due to different alleles.

Amygdala: The part of the brain whose primary role is in the formation and storage of memories associated with emotional events (such as fear and anger).

Anhedonia: The inability to experience pleasure from activities that usually produce pleasurable feelings.

Anorexia nervosa: An eating disorder characterized by a misperception of body image. Patients with anorexia nervosa often believe they are overweight even when they are grossly underweight and take extreme measures to lose weight, including restricting exercise and extreme exercise, often putting themselves at serious physical harm.

Antipsychotic: A type of drug used to treat psychosis. This class of drugs is frequently used in conditions such as schizophrenia, mania, and delusional disorder. Furthermore, because antipsychotics also have some effects as mood stabilizers, they are sometimes used in treating mood disorders.

Attachment: The emotional connection that infants and children develop toward their parents and others who care for them.

Augmentation: The practice of adding another medication to enhance the effects of the first medication.

Comorbidity: The presence of coexisting illnesses that occur together with the targeted diagnosis. Comorbidity may adversely affect the ability of affected people to function and may complicate their overall treatment plan.

Cyclothymia: Characterized by repetitive periods of mild depression followed by periods of normal or slightly elevated mood.

Delusion: A false belief based on incorrect inferences about the external reality that is firmly believed despite what almost everyone else believes and despite obvious proof or evidence to the contrary. Also, the belief is not one ordinarily accepted by other members of the person's culture or faith.

Dissociation: A psychological state in which certain thoughts, emotions, sensations, or memories are separated from the rest of a person's experience. During a dissociative episode, these thoughts, emotions, and memories are not associated with other current information as they normally would be. A dissociative episode generally serves to create a temporary mental escape from the fear and pain of a traumatic recollection and at times may lead to a complete loss of memory of the traumatic event.

Dopamine: A neurotransmitter that regulates movement, emotion, attention, motivation, and feelings of pleasure.

Etiology: The causes or origins of a medial or psychiatric disorder.

Flashback: The recurrence of a memory, feeling, or perceptual experience from the past. The past event would generally have elicited powerful feelings and emotions.

GABA: A neurotransmitter responsible for slowing down the brain. Drugs that act to increase GABA are used as anti-anxiety drugs and anti-seizure drugs.

Hallucination: A false sensory experience (can effect sight, smell, taste, touch, and hearing) that has no external stimulus. Typically, patients describe seeing things or hearing things that others cannot see or hear.

Hippocampus: The part of the brain that is critical for declarative memory; that is, the memory of persons, places, and things.

Methylphenidate: A stimulant drug used to treat ADHD. This is the generic name of Ritalin.

Neuroleptic: A synonym for antipsychotic.

Neurotransmitter: A chemical that transmits signals between the nerve cells and the brain.

Norepinephrine: A neurotransmitter found mainly in areas of the brain that are involved in governing autonomic nervous system activity, especially blood pressure and heart rate, and the flight-or-fight response.

Obsessions: Recurrent and persistent thoughts, impulses, or images experienced as intrusive and distressing. They are recognized as being excessive and unreasonable, although they are recognized as the product of one's mind and they cannot be expunged by logic or reasoning.

Panic attacks: Episodes of severe anxiety associated with symptoms such as shortness of breath, heart palpitations, chest pain, sweating, nausea, dizziness, light-headedness, and hyperventilation. During a panic attack, sufferers often believe they are dying, going insane, or having a heart attack.

Positron emission tomography: A type of brain scan that can be used to monitor the brain's activity and detect abnormalities in how it works.

Prefrontal cortex: A part of the frontal lobes of the brain that is used in planning complex cognitive behaviors, personality expression, and evaluating correct social behavior.

Psychoanalysis: A form of psychotherapy based on the psychoanalytic theory of Sigmund Freud. The most fundamental concept of psychoanalysis is the notion of the unconscious mind as a reservoir of repressed memories of traumatic events, which continuously influence conscious thought and behavior.

Psychotic: Although there are a few different definitions for this term, in this book, it is used to mean delusions, hallucinations, paranoia, and severely bizarre behavior.

Risk factors: Biological, genetic, developmental, and environmental exposures that increase the chance of developing an illness.

Serotonin: A neurotransmitter that affects emotions, behavior, and thought.

Trephination: A form of surgery in which a hole is drilled into the skull, leaving the membrane around the brain intact.

Bibliography

BOOKS

Alexander FG, Selesnick ST. 1966. *The History of Psychiatry: An Evaluation of Psychiatric Thought and Practice from Prehistoric Times to the Present*. Harper and Row.

Applewhite A, Frothingham A, Evans T. 1992. *And I Quote*. St. Martin's Press.

Beardslee WR. 2002. *Out of the Darkened Room—When a Parent Is Depressed: Protecting the Children and Strengthening the Family*. Little, Brown.

Bradbury R. 1953. *Fahrenheit 451*. Ballantine Books.

Campbell R. 1952. *Poems of Baudelaire*. Pantheon Books.

Capote T. 1987. *Answered Prayers: The Unfinished Novel*. Random House.

Carnegie D. 2004. *How to Stop Worrying and Start Living*, rev. ed. Simon and Schuster.

Diagnostic and Statistical Manual of Mental Disorders. 1994. 4th ed. American Psychiatric Association.

Dukakis K, Tye L. 2006. *Shock: The Healing Power of Electroconvulsive Therapy*. Penguin.

Forster ES. 1984. *The Complete Works of Aristotle*, vol. 2 (Barnes J., ed.). Princeton University Press.

Fry WF, Salameh WA. 1993. *Handbook of Humor and Psychotherapy*. Professional Resources Press.

Gelder M, Gath D, Mayou R. 1989. *Oxford Textbook of Psychiatry*, 2nd ed. Oxford University Press.

Gilbert P. 1992. *Depression: The Evolution of Powerlessness*. Lawrence Erlbaum Associates.

Gold M. 1986. *The Good News about Depression*. Bantam Books.

Goldsmith SK. 2002. *Reducing Suicide: A National Imperative*. National Academy Press.

Goode CT. 1972. *Byron as Critic*. B. Franklin.

Guest J. 1976. *Ordinary People*. Viking Press.

Haas EF. 1999. *Beyond the Blues: Treating Depression One Day at a Time*. Infinity Publishing.

Hayley W, Cowper W, Cunningham JW. 1851. *The Works of William Cowper: His Life, Letters, and Poems*. R. Carter & Brothers.

Hemingway E. 2003. *Ernest Hemingway: Selected Letters, 1917–1961* (Baker C, ed.). Scribner.

Houshmand Z, Livingston RB, Wallace BA. 1999. *Consciousness at the Crossroads: Conversations with the Dalai Lama on Brain Science and Buddhism*. Snow Lion Publications.

Jackson SW. 1986. *Melancholia and Depression: From Hippocratic Times to Modern Times*. Yale University Press.

Jamison KR. 1993. *Touched with Fire: Manic-Depressive Illness and the Artistic Temperament*. Free Press.

Jamison KR. 1997. *An Unquiet Mind: A Memoir of Moods and Madness*. Vintage Books.

Jamison KR. 2001. *Night Falls Fast: Understanding Suicide*. Picador.

Kessler R. 1997. *The Sins of the Father: Joseph P. Kennedy and the Dynasty He Founded*. Warner Books.

Ludwig A. 1995. *The Price of Greatness: Resolving the Creativity and Madness Controversy*. Guilford Press.

Mellow JR. 1993. *Hemingway: A Life Without Consequences*, new ed. Addison Wesley.

Milne AA. 1981. *Winnie the Pooh*. Dell Books for Young Readers.

Motion A. 1999. *Keats*. University of Chicago Press.

Nesse RM, Williams GC. 1994. *Why We Get Sick: The New Science of Darwinian Medicine*. Vintage Books.

Oates JC. 2001. *The Best American Essays of the Century*. Houghton Mifflin.

O'Connor R. 1997. *Undoing Depression: What Therapy Doesn't Teach You and Medication Can't Give You and Active Treatment of Depression*. Little, Brown.

Palahniuk C. 1999. *Survivor: A Novel*. W. W. Norton.

Pine J (ed.). 2002. *American Presidents' Wit and Wisdom: A Book of Quotations*. Dover Publications.

Quinnett P. 1993. *Suicide: The Forever Decision—for Those Thinking About Suicide, and for Those Who Know, Love, or Counsel Them*. Crossroad/Herder & Herder.

Radden J. 2000. *The Nature of Melancholy. From Aristotle to Kristeva*. Oxford University Press.

Rodriguez R. 2006. *The 1950s' Most Wanted: The Top 10 Book of Rock & Roll Rebels, Cold War Crises, and All American Oddities*. Potomac Books.

Rowe D. 1983. *Depression: The Way Out of Your Prison*. Routledge.

Saabiq S. 1991. *Fiqh-us-Sunnah*, new ed. American Trust Publications.

Sheffield A. 2003. *Depression Fallout: The Impact of Depression on Couples and What You Can Do to Preserve the Bond*. Quill/HarperCollins.

Shenk JW. 2005. *Lincoln's Melancholy: How Depression Challenged a President and Fueled His Greatness*. Houghton Mifflin.

Shields B. 2005. *Down Came the Rain: My Journey through Postpartum Depression*. Hyperion.

Solomon A. 2001. *The Noonday Demon: An Atlas of Depression*. Scribner.

Spiegel AD. 2002. *A. Lincoln, Esquire: A Shrewd, Sophisticated Lawyer in His Time.* Mercer University Press.

Stanton S. 2003. *The Tombstone Tourist: Musicians.* Simon and Schuster.

Stoll A. 2001. *The Omega-3 Connection: The Groundbreaking Anti-Depression Diet and Brain Program.* Free Press.

Styron W. 1990. *Darkness Visible.* Random House.

Szasz TS. 2006. *My Madness Saved Me: The Madness and Marriage of Virginia Woolf.* Transaction Publishers.

Thomas, GO. 1935. *William Cowper and the Eighteenth Century.* I. Nicholson and Watson.

Twain M. 1998. *Bite-Size Twain: Wit and Wisdom from the Literary Legend* (Pynchon Y, ed.). St. Martin's Press.

VanderHeyden C. 2003. *A Touch of Class.* Trafford.

Vaughn E. 2007. *Time Peace: Living Here and Now with a Timeless God.* Zondervan.

Waithe ME. 1994. *A History of Women Philosophers,* vol. 4: *Contemporary Women Philosophers, 1900–Today.* Springer.

Wolpert L. 2000. *Malignant Sadness: The Anatomy of Depression.* Free Press.

Wurtzel E. 1995. *Prozac Nation.* Riverhead Trade.

ARTICLES

Abernethy AD, Chang HT, Seidlitz L, Evinger JS, Duberstein PR. 2002. Religious coping and depression among spouses of people with lung cancer. *Psychosomatics* 43:456–463.

Airan RD, Meltzer LA, Roy M, Roy M, Gong Y, Chen H, Deisseroth K. 2007. High-speed imaging reveals neurophysiological links to behavior in an animal model of depression. *Science* 317:819–823.

Barbee EL 1992. African-American women and depression: a review and critique of the literature. *Archives of Psychiatric Nursing* 6:257–265.

Bennett AE. 1938. Convulsive (Pentamethylenetetrazol) shock therapy in depressive psychoses. Preliminary reports of results obtained in ten cases. *Acta Psychiatrica Scandinavica* 196:420.

Bennett AE. 1939. Metrazol convulsive shock therapy in affective psychoses: follow-up report of results obtained in 61 depressive and 9 manic cases. *Acta Psychiatrica Scandinavica* 198:695.

Berndt ER, Koran LM, Finkelstein SN, Gelenberg AJ, Kornstein SG, Miller IM, Thase ME, Trapp GE, Keller MB. 2000. Lost human capital from early-onset chronic depression. *American Journal of Psychiatry* 157:940–947.

Berry D. 2002. Does religious psychotherapy improves anxiety and depression in religious adults? *International Journal Psychiatric Nursing Research* 8:875–890.

Brown DR. 1990. Depression among blacks: an epidemiological perspective. In: *Handbook of Mental Health and Mental Disorder among Black Americans* (Ruiz DS, Comer JP, eds.). Greenwood Press.

Caspi A, Sugden K, Moffitt TE, Taylor A, Craig IW, Harrington H, McClay J, Mill J, Martin J, Braithwaite A, Poulton R. 2003. Influence of life stress on depression: moderation by a polymorphism in the 5-HTT gene. *Science* 301:386–389.

Froeschner EH. 1992. Two examples of ancient skull surgery. *Journal of Neurosurgery* 76:550–552.

Goldberg IK. 1980. L-tyrosine in depression. *Lancet* 2:364.

Grotjahn M. 1939 Psychiatric observations in a case of involutional melancholia treated with metrazol. *Bulletin of the Menninger Clinic* 3:122.

Guarnaccia PJ, De La Cancela V, Carrillo E. 1989. The multiple meanings of ataques de nervios in the Latino community. *Medical Anthropology* 11:47–62.

Hibbeln JR. 1998. Fish consumption and major depression. *Lancet* 351:1213.

Hodge DR. 2007. A systematic review of the empirical literature on intercessory prayer. *Research on Social Work Practice* 17:174–187.

Jamison KR. 1995. Manic-depressive illness and creativity. *Scientific American* 272:62–67.

Kartsounis LD, Poynton A, Bridges PK, Bartlett JR. 1991. Neuropsychological correlates of stereotactic subcaudate tractotomy. A prospective study. *Brain* 114:2657–2673.

Koenig HG, George LK, Peterson BL. 1998. Religiosity and remission of depression in medically ill older patients. *American Journal of Psychiatry* 155:536–542.

Lehtinen V, Joukama M, Lathela K, Raitasalo R, Jyrkinen E, Maatela J, Aromaa A. 1990. Prevalence of mental disorders among adults in Finland: basic results from the Mini-Finland Health Survey. *Acta Psychiatrica Scandinavica* 81:418–425.

Lindeman S, Hämäläinen J, Isometsä E, Kaprio J, Poikolainen K, Heikkinen M, Aro H. 2000. The 12-month prevalence and risk factors for major depressive episode: representative sample of 5993 adults. *Acta Psychiatrica Scandinavica* 102:178–184.

Link BG, Struening EL, Neese-Todd S, Asmussen S, Phelan JC. 2001. Stigma as a barrier to recovery: the consequences of stigma for the self-Esteem of people with mental illnesses. *Psychiatric Services* 52:1621–1626.

Lowry CA, Hollis JH, de Vries A, Pan B, Brunet LR, Hunt JR, Paton JF, van Kampen E, Knight DM, Evans AK, Rook GA, Lightman SL. 2007. Identification of an immune-responsive mesolimbocortical serotonergic system: potential role in regulation of emotional behavior. *Neuroscience* 146:756–772.

Nasir LS, Al-Qutob R. 2005. Barriers to the diagnosis and treatment of depression in Jordan. A Nationwide Qualitative Study. *The Journal of the American Board of Family Practice* 18:125–131.

Okello ES, Ekblad S. 2006. Lay concepts of depression among the Baganda of Uganda: a pilot Study. *Transcultural Psychiatry* 43:287–313.

Okello ES, Musisi S. 2006. Depression as a clan illness (Ebyekika) in Uganda. *World Cultural Psychiatry Research Review* 1:60–73.

Paddock S, Laje G, Charney D, Rush JA, Wilson AF, Sorant AJM, Lipsky R, Wisniewski SR, Manji H, McMahon FJ. 2007. Association of GRIK4 with outcome of antidepressant treatment in the STAR*D cohort. *American Journal of Psychiatry* 164:8.

Patel V, Abas M, Broadhead J, Todd C, Reeler A. 2001. Depression in developing countries: lessons from Zimbabwe. *British Medical Journal* 322:482–484.

Perlick DA, Rosenheck RA, Clarkin JF, Sirey JA, Salahi J, Struening EL, Link BG. 2001. Stigma as a barrier to recovery: adverse effects of perceived stigma on social adaptation of persons diagnosed with bipolar affective disorder. *Psychiatric Services* 52:1627–1632.

Pezawas L, Meyer-Lindenberg A, Drabant EM, Verchinski BA, Munoz KE, Kolachana BS, Egan MF, Mattay VS, Hariri AR, Weinberger DR. 2005. 5-HTTLPR polymorphism impacts human cingulate–amygdala interactions: a genetic susceptibility mechanism for depression. *Nature Neuroscience* 8:828–834.

Ponza G. 1876. Influence de la lumiere coloree dans le traitement de la folie. Series 5. *The Medical-Psychological Annals.* 15:20.

Rose AJ, Carlson W, Waller EM. 2007. Prospective associations of co-rumination with friendship and emotional adjustment: Considering the socioemotional trade-offs of co-rumination. *Developmental Psychology* 4:1019–1031.

Salaycik KJ, Kelly-Hayes M, Beiser A. 2007. Depressive symptoms and risk of stroke. The Framingham Study. *Stroke* 38:16–21.

Salgado de Snyder VN, Diaz-Perez MJ, Ojeda VD. 2000. The prevalence of nervios and associated symptomatology among inhabitants of Mexican rural communities. *Culture Medicine and Psychiatry* 24:453–470.

Schaefer C. 2002. Effects of laughing, smiling, and howling on mood. *Psychological Reports.* 9:1079–1080.

Stewart WF, Ricci JA, Chee E, Hahn SR, Morganstein D. 2003. Cost of lost productive work time among U.S. workers with depression. *Journal of the American Medical Association.* 289:3135–3144.

Stone JL, Miles ML. 1990. Skull trepanation among the early Indians of Canada and the United States. *Neurosurgery* 26:1015–1020.

Wang PS, Beck AL, Berglund P, McKenas DK, Pronk NP, Simon GE, Kessler RC. 2004. Effects of major depression on moment-in-time work performance. *American Journal of Psychiatry* 161:1885–1891.

Warren BJ. 1994. Depression in African-American women. *Journal of Psychosocial Nursing* 32:29–33.

Waza K, Graham AV, Zyzanski SJ, Inoue K. 1999. Comparison of symptoms in Japanese and American depressed primary care patients. *Family Practice* 16:528–533.

Wehr TA, Rosenthal NE. 1989. Seasonality and affective illness. American Journal of Psychiatry 146:829.

Weissman MM, Bland RC, Canino GJ, Faravelli C, Greenwald S, Hwu HG, Joyce PR, Karam EG, Lee CK, Lellouch J, Lepine J, Newman SC, Rubio-Stipec M, Wells JE, Wickramaratne PJ, Wittchen H, Yeh EK. 1996. Cross-national epidemiology of major depression and bipolar disorder. *Journal of the American Medical Association* 276:293–299.

Whisman M, Uebelacker LA, Weinstock, LM. 2004. Psychopathology and marital satisfaction: the importance of evaluating both partners. *Journal of Consulting and Clinical Psychology* 72:830–838.

Zhang X, Beaulieu JM, Sotnikova TD, Gainetdinov RR, Caron MG. 2004. Tryptophan hydroxylase-2 controls brain serotonin synthesis. *Science* 305:217.

OTHER CITATIONS

Berk LS. 2006. *Beta-Endorphin and HGH Increase Are Associated with Both the Anticipation and Experience of Mirthful Laughter,* Poster and paper presented at the meeting of the American Physiological Society, Behavioral Neuroscience and Drug Abuse Section, April, San Francisco, California.

Cheechoo C. 2006. *The Seventh Generation Helping to Heal: Nishnawbe Aski Youth and the Suicide Epidemic.* http://www.voicesforchildren.ca/report-Jun2006-1.htm.

An Extract of the Letter of Mr. Denis . . . Touching the Transfusion of Blood, of April 2, 1667. 1667. Philosophical Transactions of the Royal Society, 1, no. 25 (May 6, 1667), 453.

French HW. 2002. *Depression Simmers in Japan's Culture of Stoicism*. *New York Times*.

Gordinier J. 1997. Interview with Van Morrison. *Entertainment Weekly*.

Herald Sun. 2006. Go straight, Stuart Appleby. Australian Associated Press.

Manson SM, Shore JH, Bloom JD. 1985. The depressive experience in American Indian communities: a challenge for psychiatric theory and diagnosis. In: *Culture and Depression: Studies in the Anthropology and Cross-Cultural Psychiatry of Affect and Disorder* (Kleinman A, Good B, eds.). University of California Press.

Morgan J. 2004. Terry Bradshaw's winning drive against depression. *USA Today*.

Nemeroff CB. 2002. Unmet needs and the neurobiology of depression. Program and abstracts of the XII World Congress of Psychiatry, August, Yokohama, Japan, Abstract SS-21-1.

Robins LN, Regier DA (eds.). 1990. *Psychiatric Disorders in America, The Epidemiologic Catchment Area Study*. Free Press.

U.S. Department of Health and Human Services. 1999. *Mental Health: A Report of the Surgeon General—Executive Summary*. Department of Health and Human Services, Substance Abuse and Mental Health Services Administration, Center for Mental Health Services, National Institutes of Health, National Institute of Mental Health.

WEB SITES

www.aath.org

www.adam-ant.net

www.familyaware.org

www.nami.org

www.nimh.nih.gov/publicat/depression.cfm

Index

Abdominal symptoms, 55
Abe, Shintaro, 131
Académie des Sciences, 15
Academy of Motion Picture and Arts, 30
Actors, 30–32, 121
Acupuncture, 114
Adaptation, 8–9
Adeel, Muhammad Zafar, 52
Adolescence, 35, 59–61
Adolescents: antidepressant adverse effects, 64–65; diagnosing of, 61–62; family of depressed, 134–35; "girl talk" by, 76–77; mothers, 116; Native American suicide, 58; selective-serotonin reuptake inhibitors, 86
Adrenaline, 111, 112. *See also* Epinephrine
Adverse drug risks: elderly antidepressant use, 68; monoamine oxidase inhibitors, 84–85; teen antidepressant use, 64

Affect, 43
African American women, 57
Age: causes of melancholy, 13; diagnoses at different, 59–68; of onset, 142. *See also* Adolescents; Children; Elderly
Air, 14–15
Akihito, Emperor of Japan, 131
Albizzia, 110
Alcohol, 71, 82, 126
Alternative medicine, 107–17; nonherbal therapies, 113–17
Alzheimer's disease, 67
American Indians. *See* Native Americans
American Psychiatric Association (APA), 4
Amino acids, 108, 110, 111, 112
Amnesia, 100
Anatomy, 36–40, 56
Ancestral depression, 8–18
Anger, 92–93

Brown, Laura, 31
Buddhism, 51–52
Bupropion, 87–88
Burton, Robert, 12–14, 23
Byron, George Gordon, Lord, 25–26

Cameron, Donald, 100
Cancer, 74, 126, 131
Cannabis, 82
Capote, Truman, 3
Capsulotomy, 106
Carbon dioxide therapy, 81
Cardiac disorders, 75
Caribbean Latinos, 59
Carnegie, Dale, 34
Caron, Marc, 71
Carrey, Jim, 89
Case histories, 17
Case history method, 17
Cash, Pat, 122
Catholic prayers, 95–96
Caudate nucleus, 105
Cause of depression, 69–78; air quality,
    14–15; black bile, 11; brain pathways,
    139–40; diet, 13–14; humoral imbal-
    ance, 10, 12; inherited, 13; Japanese,
    55; spirits, 8–10, 53; supernatural and
    natural, 12–13; unemployment, 15
Cause of disease, 137–39
Cause of mental illness: biological/meta-
    bolic factors, 18; disease classification,
    17; impulse/conscience conflicts, 18
Cavett, Dick, 100
Celexa, 86, 141
Cell death, 140–41
Central Intelligence Agency, 100
Cerletti, Ugo, 99
Charlie Brown, 4–5, 142
Cheechoo, Catherine, 57
Chemical imbalance, 36, 70, 141
Chemistry of brain, 36–40
Chiarugi, Vincenzo, 16
Childbirth, 35, 48, 130

Childhood, 69
Children: diagnosing, 60; family of, 134–
    35; immune system, 139; Native
    American suicide, 58; parental depres-
    sion and, 133–34; prevalence in, 62–
    63; selective-serotonin reuptake inhib-
    itors, 86; storytelling, 117; as suicide
    deterrence, 122, 124; temperament
    and diet, 13
Chinese, 55–57
Choler, 12
Christie, Agatha, 23
Chronic medical illness, 70, 73–75
Cingulotomy, 105–6
Circulation, 15, 67
Citalopram, 86, 141
Clemens, Samuel Langhorne. *See* Twain,
    Mark
Cleopatra, 102
Clinical depression, 1, 6, 8, 116–17;
    chronic medical illness complication,
    73–74; prayer and faith, 116–17; twin
    studies, 70–71
Clinical histories, 40–41
Cobain, Kurt, 121, 123
Cocaine, 83
Coffee, 82
Coga, Arthur, 16
Cognitive ability, 34, 44; decline as
    cause of depression, 73; elderly
    depression, 67
Cognitive behavioral therapy (CBT),
    91–92
Collymore, Stan, 127–28
Comic strips, 4–5
Communication: antidepressant use, 86;
    interpersonal therapy, 90–91; nerve
    cells, 39, 77; parent-child, 133–34
Co-morbidity, 2–3
Companionship, 68
Complications of depression, 119–35
Composers, 121
Computerized tomography (CAT) scan, 45

About the Author

BLAISE A. AGUIRRE, M.D., is a board-certified psychiatrist and clinical instructor of psychiatry at Harvard University School of Medicine. He is the director of the Adolescent Dialectic Behavior Therapy Treatment Center at McLean Hospital in Belmont, Massachusetts. He has been a staff psychiatrist at McLean since 2000 and has been recognized for his work in the treatment of mood and personality disorders in adolescents.